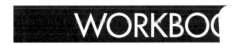

WORKBOO

INTRODUCTION TO
Medical Terminology

SECOND EDITION

MW00838086

Publisher
The Goodheart-Willcox Company, Inc.
Tinley Park, IL
www.g-w.com

Copyright © 2023
by
The Goodheart-Willcox Company, Inc.

All rights reserved. No part of this work may be reproduced, stored, or transmitted
in any form or by any electronic or mechanical means, including information storage
and retrieval systems, without the prior written permission of
The Goodheart-Willcox Company, Inc.

ISBN 978-1-64925-325-5

5 6 7 8 9 – 23 – 26 25 24

The Goodheart-Willcox Company, Inc. Brand Disclaimer: Brand names, company names, and illustrations for products and services included in this text are provided for educational purposes only and do not represent or imply endorsement or recommendation by the author or the publisher.

The Goodheart-Willcox Company, Inc. Safety Notice: The reader is expressly advised to carefully read, understand, and apply all safety precautions and warnings described in this book or that might also be indicated in undertaking the activities and exercises described herein to minimize risk of personal injury or injury to others. Common sense and good judgment should also be exercised and applied to help avoid all potential hazards. The reader should always refer to the appropriate manufacturer's technical information, directions, and recommendations; then proceed with care to follow specific equipment operating instructions. The reader should understand these notices and cautions are not exhaustive.

The publisher makes no warranty or representation whatsoever, either expressed or implied, including but not limited to equipment, procedures, and applications described or referred to herein, their quality, performance, merchantability, or fitness for a particular purpose. The publisher assumes no responsibility for any changes, errors, or omissions in this book. The publisher specifically disclaims any liability whatsoever, including any direct, indirect, incidental, consequential, special, or exemplary damages resulting, in whole or in part, from the reader's use or reliance upon the information, instructions, procedures, warnings, cautions, applications, or other matter contained in this book. The publisher assumes no responsibility for the activities of the reader.

The Goodheart-Willcox Company, Inc. Internet Disclaimer: The Internet resources and listings in this Goodheart-Willcox Publisher product are provided solely as a convenience to you. These resources and listings were reviewed at the time of publication to provide you with accurate, safe, and appropriate information. Goodheart-Willcox Publisher has no control over the referenced websites and, due to the dynamic nature of the Internet, is not responsible or liable for the content, products, or performance of links to other websites or resources. Goodheart-Willcox Publisher makes no representation, either expressed or implied, regarding the content of these websites, and such references do not constitute an endorsement or recommendation of the information or content presented. It is your responsibility to take all protective measures to guard against inappropriate content, viruses, or other destructive elements.

Cover Image Credits. Heart: first vector trend/Shutterstock.com; Brain: Veleri/Shutterstock.com; Lungs: first vector trend/Shutterstock.com.

Contents

CHAPTER 1 — Basics of Medical Terminology

Activity A   Understanding Word Parts

Review

Instructions: *Answer the following questions.*

1. What standard word parts make up most medical terms?

   _____

2. From which two languages do most medical terms derive?

   _____

3. What is the most commonly used combining vowel?

   _____

4. In general, when is a combining vowel *not* used?

   _____

5. The terms *dissect* and *dissection* are used several times in chapter 1. What do these terms mean? You may need to use a general dictionary or a medical dictionary to find their meanings.

   _____

6. What do medical terms ending in the letter combination *ae* signify?

   _____

Plural Form Terms

Instructions: *Choose the correct plural form of each of the following terms.*

1. _____ appendix
   A. appendixes
   B. appendices
   C. appendicae
   D. appendicies

2. _____ index
   A. indexaces
   B. indexi
   C. indexes
   D. indices

3. _____ atrium
   A. atria
   B. atriumes
   C. atrium
   D. atriumies

Copyright Goodheart-Willcox Co., Inc.
May not be reproduced or posted to a publicly accessible website.

4. _____ bronchus
    A. bronchae
    B. bronchuses
    C. bronchi
    D. bronchies

Word Parts Matching, Part 1

Instructions: *Match each of the following word parts with the correct meaning.*

1. _____ a-, an-

2. _____ -algia

3. _____ hyper-

4. _____ -itis

5. _____ trans-

6. _____ inter-

7. _____ -pathy

8. _____ peri-

9. _____ -oma

10. _____ –ial

A. inflammation

B. between

C. across

D. pain

E. around; surrounding

F. not; without

G. tumor; mass

H. above; above normal; excessive

I. disease

J. pertaining to

Word Parts Matching, Part 2

Instructions: *Match each of the following word parts with the correct meaning.*

1. _____ cervic/o

2. _____ path/o

3. _____ gastr/o

4. _____ cost/o

5. _____ cephal/o

6. _____ arthr/o

7. _____ my/o

8. _____ lip/o

9. _____ hem/o

10. _____ nas/o

A. rib

B. muscle

C. blood

D. disease

E. fat

F. neck; cervix (neck of uterus)

G. head

H. stomach

I. joint

J. nose

Copyright Goodheart-Willcox Co., Inc.
May not be reproduced or posted to a publicly accessible website.

Name _____

Activity B   Case Study—Medical Records and Abbreviations

Instructions: *Read the case study on page 2 of your textbook, and then define each of the following abbreviations.*

Example

CBC: complete blood count

1. UA: _____

2. EKG: _____

3. CXR: _____

4. Pt: _____

5. NPO: _____

6. pre-op: _____

7. postop: _____

8. VS: _____

9. c/o: _____

10. abd: _____

11. SOB: _____

12. OB/GYN: _____

13. STAT: _____

14. b.i.d.: _____

15. Explain why healthcare organizations might use military time for their records.

    _____

    _____

    _____

    _____

Copyright Goodheart-Willcox Co., Inc.
May not be reproduced or posted to a publicly accessible website.

Terms Related to Diseases, Conditions, and Assessment

Review

Instructions: *Answer the following questions.*

1. Explain the difference between the terms *condition* and *disease*.

   _____

   _____

2. What is a nonmalignant and noncancerous tumor considered to be?

   _____

3. What is an abnormal growth, even if it is noncancerous, called?

   _____

4. What type of stroke is caused by a temporary deficiency in blood flow to the brain?

   _____

5. What type of disease is inherited from one's biological parents?

   _____

6. What disease has a weakening or fatiguing effect?

   _____

7. What infection is acquired in a hospital setting that was not present upon admission?

   _____

8. What is the widespread outbreak of a disease that occurs within a population, group, or area of land?

   _____

9. What is a condition that occurs as a complication of medical or surgical intervention, such as hair loss after chemotherapy for cancer treatment, called?

   _____

10. What is the time period of recovery after an illness or injury called?

   _____

11. What is a pathogen that normally does not cause disease in healthy people but may cause someone with a weakened immune system to get sick called?

   _____

12. A disease that does not have any known cause is called what type of condition?

   _____

13. What condition occurs because of an external factor, such as trauma or an airborne virus?

   _____

Copyright Goodheart-Willcox Co., Inc.
May not be reproduced or posted to a publicly accessible website.

14. What disorder is a condition that is present at birth?

_____

15. What is a set of signs or symptoms that occur together as part of a disease process?

_____

Matching

Instructions: *Match each of the following terms with the correct meaning.*

1. _____ the use of smell to detect abnormalities

2. _____ clinical presentation

3. _____ the use of pressure on the skin above internal organs or structures

4. _____ objective observations

5. _____ the process of listening to body sounds using a stethoscope

6. _____ prediction of the probable outcome of a condition

7. _____ the use of lab tests, X-rays, and other diagnostic tools to identify a condition

8. _____ a patient's awareness of abnormalities or discomfort

9. _____ the process of observing one or more areas of the body

10. _____ tapping on surface areas of the body to produce a vibrating sound

A. auscultation

B. diagnostic testing

C. inspection

D. manifestation

E. olfaction

F. palpation

G. percussion

H. prognosis

I. signs

J. symptoms

Copyright Goodheart-Willcox Co., Inc.
May not be reproduced or posted to a publicly accessible website.

Chapter 1 Practice Test

Review

Instructions: *Answer the following questions.*

1. The most basic units that combine to make a medical term are called what?

   _____

2. What is a root word plus a combining vowel?

   _____

3. What is something helpful you can do with terms to learn medical terms?

   _____

4. What is the study of the causes of pathological conditions?

   _____

5. What is a shortened form of a medical term or phrase?

   _____

Definitions, Part 1

Instructions: *Using the word parts on pages 6–8 of your textbook, define the following medical terms.*

1. gastritis: _____

2. lipoma: _____

3. biologist: _____

4. thoracotomy: _____

5. hepatomegaly: _____

Definitions, Part 2

Instructions: *Using the word parts on pages 6–8 of your textbook, identify the medical term that corresponds to each of the following definitions.*

1. a microorganism that produces disease: _____

2. a condition in which there is too much sugar in the blood: _____

3. a tumor of the connective tissue: _____

Copyright Goodheart-Willcox Co., Inc.
May not be reproduced or posted to a publicly accessible website.

Medical Record Interpretation

Instructions: *Read the following medical record and then identify the meaning of the abbreviations that appear in bold and are listed after the record. Refer to the table on pages 13–14 and Appendix B on pages 480–484 of your textbook.*

Medical Record

A 6 **y/o AAF** presents to **ER** with **c/o SOB** and wheezing on inspiration. Pt's caregiver states that she has had symptoms for several days and that symptoms have progressively worsened in the past 12 hours. **Pt** has a history of asthma. Caregiver reports that she has not been using her asthma medications for the past week because they "did not have the money to buy the medicine."

Assessment: Well developed, alert, and responsive. **wt**: 50 lbs; **ht**: 42 inches. **V/S WNL. NKDA.**

Orders: **STAT CXR**, **CBC. Consult** with Pediatric Pulmonologist and Social Services for assistance with asthma medication cost.

1. y/o: _____
2. AAF: _____
3. ER: _____
4. c/o: _____
5. SOB: _____
6. Pt: _____
7. wt: _____
8. ht: _____
9. V/S: _____
10. WNL: _____
11. NKDA: _____
12. STAT: _____
13. CXR: _____
14. CBC: _____
15. Consult: _____

Time Conversion, Part 1

Instructions: *Convert the following standard times to military time.*

1. 1:15 p.m.: _____
2. 1:15 a.m.: _____
3. 10:45 p.m.: _____

Time Conversion, Part 2

Instructions: *Convert the following military times to standard time.*

1. 2100: _____
2. 1330: _____

Copyright Goodheart-Willcox Co., Inc.
May not be reproduced or posted to a publicly accessible website.

Notes

_____

_____

_____

_____

_____

_____

_____

_____

_____

_____

_____

_____

_____

_____

_____

_____

_____

_____

_____

_____

_____

_____

_____

_____

_____

_____

_____

_____

_____

_____

_____

Copyright Goodheart-Willcox Co., Inc.
May not be reproduced or posted to a publicly accessible website.

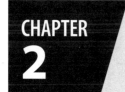

Basics of the Body

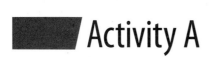 Activity A   Anatomy and Physiology: Descriptive Terms

Review

Instructions: *Answer the following question.*

1. Explain the difference between the terms *anatomy* and *physiology.*

_____

_____

_____

_____

_____

_____

Term Identification

Instructions: *Identify the correct terms in the following paragraph.*

   The body is considered to be in the anatomical position when a person is standing **[Term 1]** with the head and feet facing **[Term 2]**, the arms at the **[Term 3]**, and the palms of the hands facing **[Term 4]**.

1. Term 1: _____

2. Term 2: _____

3. Term 3: _____

4. Term 4: _____

Matching

Instructions: *Match each of the following body positions with the correct description.*

1. _____ sitting position, head of bed elevated

2. _____ lying flat with the face down

3. _____ left or right side; lying position

4. _____ normal standing position

5. _____ lying flat with the face up

6. _____ lying facedown with knees bent while resting on the knees and chest

7. _____ lying on side with hip and knee straight, and the other hip and knee bent or flexed

A. erect

B. supine

C. prone

D. high Fowler's

E. Sims'

F. lateral

G. knee-chest

Copyright Goodheart-Willcox Co., Inc.
May not be reproduced or posted to a publicly accessible website.

Labeling

Instructions: *Label the three planes in the following image.*

1. Item 1:_____

2. Item 2:_____

3. Item 3:_____

Body Cavity Labeling

Instructions: *The body cavities are cranial, thoracic, abdominal, and pelvic. For each of the following organs, indicate the body cavity in which it is located. You will use some body cavities more than once.*

1. heart: _____

2. stomach: _____

3. brain:_____

4. urinary bladder:_____

5. lungs: _____

6. uterus: _____

7. gallbladder: _____

1.

2.

3.

© *Body Scientific International*

Review

Instructions: *Answer the following questions.*

1. How would an anatomist (someone who is a specialist in the study of the structure of the body) define the term *hypochondriac*?

   _____

   _____

   _____

   _____

2. Where is the epigastric region located?

   _____

   _____

   _____

   _____

3. What does the term *hypogastric* mean?

   _____

   _____

   _____

   _____

Copyright Goodheart-Willcox Co., Inc.
May not be reproduced or posted to a publicly accessible website.

◢ Activity B   Body Organization

Review

Instructions: *Answer the following questions.*

1. Which term describes a state of physiological balance in the body?

   _____

2. Which term is used to describe the study of cells?

   _____

3. What is the "controlling" structure of the cell?

   _____

4. Which term describes a positive-charge ion?

   _____

5. Which term describes a negative-charge ion?

   _____

6. Define *pH*.

   _____

Matching

Instructions: *Match each of the following cell types with the correct description.*

1. _____ contains large, empty spaces

2. _____ long, with several fibrous extensions

3. _____ long and slender

4. _____ flat and square

A. muscle cells
B. epithelial cells
C. fat cells
D. nerve cells

Muscle Types

Instructions: *Answer the following questions about types of muscle.*

1. What are the three types of muscle cells?

   _____

2. Which type of muscle attaches to bone?

   _____

3. Which type of muscle is found in the heart?

   _____

4. Which type of muscle is found in the walls of hollow organs, such as the intestines?

   _____

Copyright Goodheart-Willcox Co., Inc.
May not be reproduced or posted to a publicly accessible website.

Labeling Body Systems

Instructions: *The major systems of the body are the integumentary system, skeletal system, muscular system, nervous system, endocrine system, respiratory system, cardiovascular system, lymphatic system, digestive system, urinary system, male reproductive system, and female reproductive system. Indicate in which body system each of the following organs is located. You will use some body systems more than once. Some organs may be in more than one system.*

1. lungs: _____

2. bones: _____

3. urinary bladder: _____

4. trachea: _____

5. spleen: _____

6. heart: _____

7. uterus: _____

8. skin: _____

9. joints: _____

10. blood vessels: _____

11. brain: _____

12. testes: _____

13. stomach: _____

14. spinal cord: _____

15. muscles: _____

16. nasal cavity: _____

17. pancreas: _____

18. lymph nodes: _____

19. kidney: _____

20. tongue: _____

21. prostate gland: _____

22. ovaries: _____

Copyright Goodheart-Willcox Co., Inc.
May not be reproduced or posted to a publicly accessible website.

Chapter 2 Practice Test

Review

Instructions: *Answer the following questions.*

1. In anatomy, the human body is divided into what three imaginary flat sections?

_____

2. What is a space within the body that contains and protects internal organs and other body structures?

_____

3. What is the basic structural unit of the body?

_____

4. What term means "the study of disease"?

_____

5. What is a structure that is composed of several kinds of tissues working together to perform a specific function?

_____

Body System Identification

Instructions: *Identify the body system that corresponds to each of the following functions.*

1. protects the body against microorganisms:

_____

2. regulates body functions:

_____

3. produces vitamin D:

_____

4. transmits sensory messages:

_____

5. filters airborne pollutants:

_____

6. protects internal organs:

_____

7. produces body heat:

_____

8. carries chemical wastes to the kidneys:

_____

9. removes solid wastes from the body:

_____

Copyright Goodheart-Willcox Co., Inc.
May not be reproduced or posted to a publicly accessible website.

10. facilitates survival of the species:

_____

11. produces red blood cells:

_____

12. filters blood to remove wastes:

_____

Body Position Identification

Instructions: *List the most commonly used body position for each of the following procedures or goals.*

1. chest X-ray:

_____

2. preventing aspiration:

_____

3. MRI scan:

_____

Abdominal Quadrant Identification

Instructions: *The abdominal quadrants are RUQ, LUQ, RLQ, and LLQ. Identify the abdominal quadrant in which each of the following organs is located.*

1. left ovary:

_____

2. stomach:

_____

3. left ureter:

_____

4. right fallopian tube:

_____

5. gallbladder:

_____

6. spleen:

_____

7. right lobe of the liver:

_____

Copyright Goodheart-Willcox Co., Inc.
May not be reproduced or posted to a publicly accessible website.

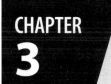

CHAPTER 3

The Integumentary System

Activity A   Understanding Word Parts

Word Parts Matching, Part 1

Instructions: *Match each of the following word parts with the correct meaning.*

1. _____ cell
2. _____ tumor; mass
3. _____ self
4. _____ full of; pertaining to; sugar
5. _____ flow; excessive discharge
6. _____ on; over; upon
7. _____ skin
8. _____ surgical removal; excision
9. _____ through
10. _____ below; under

A. epi-
B. -ectomy
C. sub-
D. -oma
E. auto-
F. -cyte
G. per-
H. -derma
I. -ose
J. -rrhea

Word Parts Matching, Part 2

Instructions: *Match each of the following word parts with the correct meaning.*

1. _____ hardening
2. _____ fat; sebum
3. _____ hair
4. _____ nail
5. _____ wrinkle
6. _____ fungus
7. _____ tissue
8. _____ dry
9. _____ eyelid
10. _____ heat; burn

A. myc/o
B. blephar/o
C. xer/o
D. rhytid/o
E. hist/o
F. scler/o
G. ungu/o
H. cauter/o
I. steat/o
J. trich/o

Copyright Goodheart-Willcox Co., Inc.
May not be reproduced or posted to a publicly accessible website.

Build the Medical Term

Instructions: *Use the combining forms and suffixes listed on pages 45–46 of your textbook to build the medical term that corresponds to each of the following definitions.*

1. Word part: lip/o

   Definition: a mass of fat

   Term: _____

2. Word part: -osis

   Definition: abnormal condition of being bluish in color

   Term: _____

3. Word part: dermat/o

   Definition: inflammation of the skin

   Term: _____

4. Word part: -derma

   Definition: condition of hardening of the skin

   Term: _____

5. Word part: -esis

   Definition: condition of profuse sweating

   Term: _____

Medical Terms and Definitions

Instructions: *Break down each of the following medical terms into its word parts (prefix, root word, combining vowel, and suffix if used). Then define each term.*

1. psoriasis

   Breakdown: _____

   Define: _____

2. immunology

   Breakdown: _____

   Define: _____

3. cryotherapy

   Breakdown: _____

   Define: _____

4. ecchymosis

   Breakdown: _____

   Define: _____

5. onychomycosis

   Breakdown: _____

   Define: _____

Copyright Goodheart-Willcox Co., Inc.
May not be reproduced or posted to a publicly accessible website.

6. steatorrhea

Breakdown: _____

Define: _____

7. melanoma

Breakdown: _____

Define: _____

8. subcutaneous

Breakdown: _____

Define: _____

9. adipose

Breakdown: _____

Define: _____

10. xeroderma

Breakdown: _____

Define: _____

Copyright Goodheart-Willcox Co., Inc.
May not be reproduced or posted to a publicly accessible website.

Activity B Interpreting Medical Records

Instructions: *Read the following medical records. Then define the abbreviations and answer the questions that follow the medical record.*

Medical Record A

A 27 **y/o** male presents to **ER** with second-degree burns to 9 percent of the lateral **RLE** as a result of a fire pit malfunction. **Tx** of the area includes irrigation with normal saline solution, applying silver sulfadiazine **oint**, and dressing the area with sterile gauze.

1. y/o: _____

2. ER: _____

3. RLE: _____

4. Tx: _____

5. oint: _____

6. Explain where the burn was located.

_____

Medical Record B

A 60 y/o female presents to outpatient cosmetic surgery center to be evaluated for a possible face-lift. **Pt** is a **NS**. Eval of **HEENT WNL**. Schedule this patient for rhytidectomy, bilateral blepharoplasty, and dermabrasion. Explain to patient that these procedures are not covered by her insurance company because they are considered cosmetic.

1. Pt: _____

2. NS: _____

3. HEENT: _____

4. WNL: _____

5. Explain the three procedures listed in this medical record in terms that the patient would understand.

_____

Medical Record C

Pt is a 52 y/o male with an **OH** of outdoor construction work. Pt was seen by **PCP** due to **c/o** a lesion on the lobe of the **AS** that "just would not heal." **Bx** of site reveals Dx of basal cell carcinoma. Pt referred to dermatologist for possible Mohs surgery.

1. OH: _____

2. PCP: _____

3. c/o: _____

4. AS: _____

5. Bx: _____

6. Describe Mohs surgery.

_____

Copyright Goodheart-Willcox Co., Inc.
May not be reproduced or posted to a publicly accessible website.

Name _____

Medical Record D

Pt has **hx** of excision of benign skin lesions, including a **cyst** in the **LLQ** of the **abd** area and a **nevus** on the R posterior lumbar area. 6-month **postop** evaluation shows the incision on the posterior lumbar area is a 2 cm x 0.2 cm well-healed cicatrix. The area on the anterior side reveals a 4 cm x 2.3 cm keloid. Pt states that this lesion is bothersome but denies pain. Recommend injecting the keloid with prednisone.

1. hx: _____

2. cyst: _____

3. LLQ: _____

4. abd: _____

5. nevus: _____

6. postop: _____

7. Explain the difference between a *cicatrix* and a *keloid*.

   _____

   _____

   _____

8. Where is this patient's keloid located?

   _____

Copyright Goodheart-Willcox Co., Inc.
May not be reproduced or posted to a publicly accessible website.

Activity C Comprehending Anatomy and Physiology Terminology

Review, Part 1

Instructions: *Answer the following questions.*

1. In its role as a physical barrier, what are three elements from which the skin protects the body?

   _____

2. Explain how the skin helps regulate the body's internal temperature.

   _____

   _____

3. What is the purpose of tactile receptors?

   _____

4. Where would you find mucous membranes in the body?

   _____

5. What does the term *stratified* mean?

   _____

6. What does the term *squamous* mean?

   _____

7. What three characteristics does connective tissue provide to the skin?

   _____

Copyright Goodheart-Willcox Co., Inc.
May not be reproduced or posted to a publicly accessible website.

Skin Structure Labeling

Instructions: *Label the skin structures in the following image.*

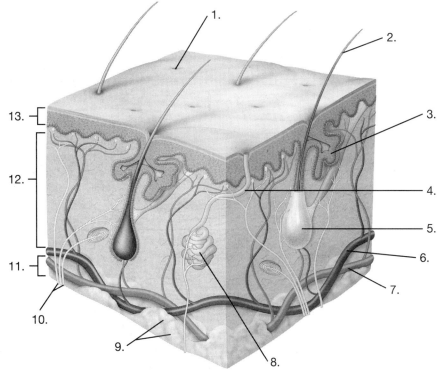

© *Body Scientific International*

1. Item 1:_____

2. Item 2:_____

3. Item 3:_____

4. Item 4:_____

5. Item 5:_____

6. Item 6:_____

7. Item 7:_____

8. Item 8:_____

9. Item 9:_____

10. Item 10:_____

11. Item 11:_____

12. Item 12:_____

13. Item 13:_____

Copyright Goodheart-Willcox Co., Inc.
May not be reproduced or posted to a publicly accessible website.

Skin Layer Labeling

Instructions: *Label the layers of skin in the following image.*

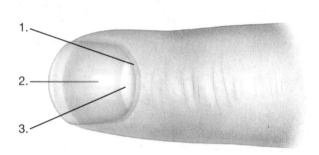
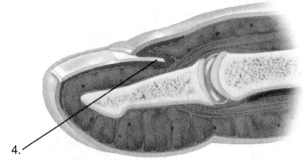

© Body Scientific International

1. Item 1:_____

2. Item 2:_____

3. Item 3:_____

4. Item 4:_____

Review, Part 2

Instructions: *Answer the following questions.*

1. Which layer of the skin contains the cells that store fat?

    _____

2. What is the major difference between sebaceous glands and sweat glands?

    _____

3. Where would you find the greatest number of sweat glands in the body?

    _____

4. Explain what causes the body odor associated with sweating.

    _____

5. On average, who has more hair follicles, people with red hair or people with blond hair?

    _____

6. What causes hair to "stand on end" when someone is frightened?

    _____

    _____

7. What substance makes up the nails?

    _____

8. Why should healthcare professionals look closely at the nails of the patients they are examining?

    _____

    _____

Copyright Goodheart-Willcox Co., Inc.
May not be reproduced or posted to a publicly accessible website.

Name _____

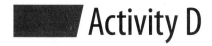 **Activity D   Understanding Terms Related to Diseases and Conditions**

Review

Instructions: *Answer the following questions.*

1. What is the difference between impetigo and tinea?

_____

_____

_____

_____

2. A possible side effect of some medications, such as prednisone, is the occurrence of round, pinpoint spots under the skin. What is the medical term for these spots?

_____

3. Which condition causes the veins, usually in the lower extremities, to lose their elasticity and appear to be twisting?

_____

4. What is the difference between a keloid and a wart?

_____

_____

_____

_____

5. How would you be able to visualize the difference between a case of psoriasis and a case of eczema?

_____

_____

6. Which chronic autoimmune condition may result in hardening of the connective tissue?

_____

7. A symptom of an allergic reaction to a food or medication may be itching and the formation of hives. What medical term describes this condition?

_____

8. Refer to the list of diseases and conditions associated with the integumentary system. Which two conditions are caused by poor blood circulation?

_____

9. How do you determine if a burn is a first- or second-degree burn?

_____

_____

_____

Copyright Goodheart-Willcox Co., Inc.
May not be reproduced or posted to a publicly accessible website.

10. How do you determine if a burn is a second- or third-degree burn?

_____

_____

_____

_____

11. When patients have burns, what do clinicians look at?

_____

_____

12. What is the percentage of total body surface area for both the anterior and posterior of the head and back?

_____

Matching

Instructions: *Match each description with the correct medical term.*

1. _____ small, raised skin lesion filled with clear fluid

2. _____ crack or groove, as in a sore

3. _____ smooth, slightly swollen area redder or paler than the surrounding skin

4. _____ open sore or erosion of the skin

5. _____ solid skin elevation with distinct borders

6. _____ small, infected skin elevation that contains pus

7. _____ closed, thick-walled sac containing fluid

8. _____ small, flat, discolored lesion

9. _____ skin elevation larger than 1 centimeter

10. _____ highly pigmented lesion

A. macula
B. papule
C. nodule
D. wheal
E. vesicle
F. nevus
G. pustule
H. fissure
I. ulcer
J. cyst

Copyright Goodheart-Willcox Co., Inc.
May not be reproduced or posted to a publicly accessible website.

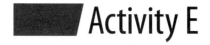 **Activity E** Understanding Diagnostic- and Treatment-Related Terms

Review

Instructions: *Answer the following questions.*

1. Explain the difference between a scratch test and an intradermal test.

   _____

   _____

   _____

   _____

2. A patient comes into the clinic with a possible basal cell carcinoma. What procedure may be performed to make sure this is the correct diagnosis?

   _____

3. The pathology report for the patient mentioned in question 2 came back as positive for basal cell carcinoma. The lesion is not very big or very deep. What might be the possible treatment to remove this cancer?

   _____

Dermatology Technician Review

Instructions: *Imagine that you are a dermatology technician in a busy clinic. Answer the following questions using information you learned in chapter 3.*

1. Your doctor is preparing to treat a young girl who has warts on her feet. Write an explanation you would give to the patient about what the doctor is going to do.

   _____

   _____

2. The next patient you are assisting the doctor with is having a cancerous growth removed from the right scapular area using the Mohs surgery technique. The patient has been prepared for the procedure, and the doctor makes the first incision before leaving the room. The patient seems worried. How will you explain what is happening to the patient?

   _____

   _____

3. Your next patient had sclerotherapy preformed a week ago. She is concerned that she cannot see a difference in her condition. How will you explain the healing process to your patient?

   _____

   _____

   _____

Copyright Goodheart-Willcox Co., Inc.
May not be reproduced or posted to a publicly accessible website.

4. In the next room, a patient is waiting to have his second treatment of debridement after suffering a third-degree burn on his left forearm. Last week, during the first treatment, the patient stated that his pain level was not as bad as he expected. However, the patient has noted that he is having more pain in the affected area, and he is concerned about the treatment today. He says he does not understand why he has to go through with this treatment today. How will you explain the purpose of this procedure?

_____

_____

5. You have relieved some of the burn patient's fears about the purpose of the debridement procedure, but he is still very apprehensive about the pain. What type of medication might the doctor give this patient prior to his procedure to help manage the pain?

_____

6. During the debridement procedure, the doctor notes an area of possible infection. What type of medication might the doctor prescribe for this patient?

_____

7. The next patient is a 4 y/o boy who has a severe rash due to poison ivy. His mother says that he cannot sleep well because he keeps waking up feeling itchy. What type of medication might the doctor prescribe for this patient?

_____

8. The next patient is a 26 y/o female who is undergoing removal of a tattoo on her posterior right shoulder area. This is her third session. What type of therapy would the doctor use for this procedure?

_____

9. Next, the doctor will be performing an excision of a squamous cell carcinoma on a 72 y/o male. The doctor tells the patient that he will have to perform an autograft procedure. When the doctor leaves the room, the patient asks you what an "autograft" is. What will you tell this patient?

_____

_____

10. Your next scheduled patient is a 15 y/o male with tinea of the feet, bilaterally. What type of medication might the doctor prescribe for this patient?

_____

11. The final patient of the day is a 55 y/o female with multiple skin tags in the neck area. What procedure will the doctor most likely perform to treat this skin condition?

_____

12. Now you have some phone calls to return. Your last call is to a patient who has sought treatment for multiple skin cancers at your clinic. Yesterday, this patient visited an orthopedic specialist because he was complaining of back pain. The patient tells you that the orthopedic specialist gave him a transdermal pain medication called Duragesic. The patient is calling your office because he does not understand what the term transdermal means. He thought that you could explain how he is supposed to use this medication. What would you tell him?

_____

_____

_____

Copyright Goodheart-Willcox Co., Inc.
May not be reproduced or posted to a publicly accessible website.

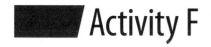 **Activity F   Preparing for Your Future in Healthcare**

Define Word Parts

Instructions: *Define the following word parts related to healthcare professions.*

1. bi/o: _____

2. dermat/o: _____

3. path/o: _____

4. -dermis: _____

5. -ectomy: _____

Define Medical Terms

Instructions: *Define the following medical terms related to healthcare professions.*

1. dermatoplasty: _____

2. hypodermic: _____

3. onychectomy: _____

Review

Instructions: *Answer the following questions using the information from the Chapter 3 Careers to Consider section of your textbook.*

1. Of the three healthcare professionals mentioned, which one requires the most education?

   _____

2. Which of these three professionals requires the least education?

   _____

3. Which of these professionals can prescribe medications?

   _____

4. Which of these professionals can perform surgery?

   _____

Healthcare Professionals

Instructions: *For each of the professionals listed, identify two or three possible facilities where the professional may work.*

1. dermatologist:

   _____

2. dermatology nurse practitioner:

   _____

3. dermatology technician:

   _____

Copyright Goodheart-Willcox Co., Inc.
May not be reproduced or posted to a publicly accessible website.

Chapter 3 Practice Test

Definitions

Instructions: *Using the word parts on pages 45–46 of your textbook, identify the medical term that corresponds to each of the following definitions.*

1. removal of a nail: _____

2. a red (blood) cell: _____

3. the study of tissues: _____

4. treatment with cold: _____

5. inflammation of the eyelid: _____

6. inflammation of a gland: _____

7. the study of cells: _____

Build Medical Terms

Instructions: *Use the following prefixes and suffixes listed on pages 45–46 to build the medical term that corresponds to each of the following definitions.*

1. Word part: -osis

   Definition: the abnormal condition of dry, scaly skin

   Term: _____

2. Word part: par-

   Definition: an abnormal feeling or sensation

   Term: _____

3. Word part: -osis

   Definition: an abnormal condition of hardening

   Term: _____

4. Word part: -ic

   Definition: pertaining to death

   Term: _____

5. Word part: -osis

   Definition: an abnormal condition of blood in the tissues

   Term: _____

Medical Terms and Definitions

Instructions: *Break down each of the following medical terms into its word parts (prefix, root word, combining vowel, and suffix if used). Then define each term.*

1. hidradenitis

   Breakdown: _____

   Define: _____

Copyright Goodheart-Willcox Co., Inc.
May not be reproduced or posted to a publicly accessible website.

2. erythematous

    Breakdown: _____

    Define: _____

3. pruritic

    Breakdown: _____

    Define: _____

4. trichomycosis

    Breakdown: _____

    Define: _____

Review

Instructions: *Answer the following questions.*

1. List the four major functions of the skin.

    _____

    _____

2. What is the term for the outermost layer of the skin?

    _____

3. What is the term for the cells that produce dark pigment in the skin?

    _____

4. Melanin is the pigment that gives skin its color. What is another important function of this pigment?

    _____

5. Which term describes the oil that is produced in the sebaceous glands and helps to lubricate the hair and skin?

    _____

6. Which term that comes from the Greek word for "glue" is used to describe the connective tissue in the skin?

    _____

7. Which term describes the layer of skin containing fat cells?

    _____

8. Which term describes the half-moon-shaped structure that is found in the nail?

    _____

Disease or Condition Identification

Instructions: *Identify the term that corresponds to each disease or condition described.*

1. a burn that results in blisters: _____

2. bacterial infection common in children that includes vesicles, pustules, and crusted-over lesions:

    _____

3. an abnormally raised and thickened scar: _____

4. hair loss: _____

Copyright Goodheart-Willcox Co., Inc.
May not be reproduced or posted to a publicly accessible website.

5. a blister: _____

6. a freckle: _____

7. a small infected area of skin that contains pus: _____

Treatment or Procedure Identification

Instructions: *Identify the term that corresponds to each treatment or procedure described.*

1. the destruction of tissue through heat, cold, or an electric current: _____

2. common treatment for the removal of basal cell tumors: _____

3. removal of damaged tissue to promote healing and prevent infections: _____

4. the procedure used to dissolve varicose veins: _____

Copyright Goodheart-Willcox Co., Inc.
May not be reproduced or posted to a publicly accessible website.

The Skeletal System

Activity A   Understanding Word Parts

Word Parts Matching, Part 1

Instructions: *Match each of the following word parts with the correct meaning.*

1. _____ within; into
2. _____ inflammation
3. _____ change; beyond
4. _____ around; surrounding
5. _____ softening
6. _____ process of cutting; incision
7. _____ pain
8. _____ between
9. _____ deficiency
10. _____ pertaining to

A. meta-
B. -algia
C. inter-
D. -itis
E. -al
F. intra-
G. -tomy
H. peri-
I. -penia
J. -malacia

Word Parts Matching, Part 2

Instructions: *Match each of the following word parts with the correct meaning.*

1. _____ joint
2. _____ wrist
3. _____ crooked; bent
4. _____ lubricating fluid of joints
5. _____ tendon
6. _____ foot; child
7. _____ bone marrow; spinal cord
8. _____ straight
9. _____ vertebra; backbone
10. _____ ankle

A. myel/o
B. arthr/o
C. ped/o
D. scoli/o
E. carp/o
F. synovi/o
G. tars/o
H. tendon/o
I. spondyl/o
J. orth/o

Copyright Goodheart-Willcox Co., Inc.
May not be reproduced or posted to a publicly accessible website.

Medical Terms and Definitions

Instructions: *Break down each of the following medical terms into its word parts (prefix, root word, combining vowel, and suffix if used). Then define each term.*

1. intercostal

   Breakdown: _____

   Define: _____

2. tendonitis

   Breakdown: _____

   Define: _____

3. kyphosis

   Breakdown: _____

   Define: _____

4. antipyretic

   Breakdown: _____

   Define: _____

5. arthralgia

   Breakdown: _____

   Define: _____

6. craniotomy

   Breakdown: _____

   Define: _____

7. arthroplasty

   Breakdown: _____

   Define: _____

8. rheumatoid

   Breakdown: _____

   Define: _____

9. subcostal

   Breakdown: _____

   Define: _____

10. lumbalgia

    Breakdown: _____

    Define: _____

11. narcosis

    Breakdown: _____

    Define: _____

Copyright Goodheart-Willcox Co., Inc.
May not be reproduced or posted to a publicly accessible website.

◢ Activity B Interpreting Medical Records

Definitions

Instructions: *Use a regular dictionary or a medical dictionary to define the following terms.*

1. aggravation

_____

_____

2. alleviate

_____

_____

3. therapeutic

_____

_____

4. bulge

_____

_____

5. In your own words, explain what *pain radiating* means.

_____

_____

6. What does the term *over-the-counter medication* mean?

_____

_____

Medical Record Interpretation

Instructions: *Read the following medical record. Then, using the chapter and Appendix B: Medical Abbreviations in the text, define the abbreviations that follow the medical record.*

Medical Record

Patient's Name: Jane Doe

ID Number: 12345

Date of Service: May 3, 20XX

Subjective Data: 45 **y/o** female with **c/o** increasing difficulty using her **R** hand. **Pt** states she is "continually dropping things like her car keys and hairbrush." Pt states symptoms have worsened over the past six months. Pt states that she wakes up in the morning with severe numbness and tingling, and that it takes approximately two to three hours for symptoms to reduce in intensity. Pt's **OH** is a computer analyst for the past 20 years. Pt states that her **PCP** has ordered **OTC NSAID**s, occupational therapy evaluation with recommendations of home exercises, and night splinting. Pt states that symptoms have worsened despite conservative **Tx**. Pt referred to orthopedics for evaluation.

Objective Data: Pt is a well-developed female. **Ht**: 65 inches. **Wt**: 154.2 pounds. **HEENT** exam **WNL**. Evaluation of affected extremity reveals slight atrophy of R forearm in relationship to the **L** side. Wrist circumference: R: 18 **cm**, **L**: 19 cm. Pt is not able to distinguish between light and firm pinpoint pressures in the 2nd to 4th digits of the R hand.

Assessment: Moderate to severe **CTS**

Plan: Order **NCV** study. If this test indicates moderate to severe CTS, schedule Pt for endoscopic R carpal tunnel release. Instruct Pt that if surgery is required, she will have to schedule to be off work for at least six weeks. If NCV study does not reveal CTS, contact Pt to return to clinic for further evaluation and Tx.

Copyright Goodheart-Willcox Co., Inc.

May not be reproduced or posted to a publicly accessible website.

1. y/o: _____

2. c/o: _____

3. R: _____

4. Pt: _____

5. OH: _____

6. PCP: _____

7. OTC: _____

8. NSAID: _____

9. Tx: _____

10. Ht: _____

11. Wt: _____

12. HEENT: _____

13. WNL: _____

14. L: _____

15. cm: _____

16. CTS: _____

17. NCV: _____

Define Medical Terms

Instructions: *Define the following terms. If you are unsure what a term means, look up the term in the Glossary/Index of your text or use a medical dictionary.*

1. orthopedics: _____

2. conservative treatment: _____

3. extremity: _____

4. digits: _____

5. endoscopy: _____

Review

Instructions: *Answer the following questions related to Jane Doe's medical record. You may need to conduct research using reliable and valid medical resources to find an answer.*

1. Why do you think the patient described in this medical record developed CTS?

_____

_____

_____

2. What are some steps that patients can take to prevent or minimize this condition?

_____

_____

_____

Copyright Goodheart-Willcox Co., Inc.
May not be reproduced or posted to a publicly accessible website.

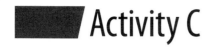 **Activity C**   Comprehending Anatomy
and Physiology Terminology

Review, Part 1

Instructions: *Answer the following questions.*

1. Explain the difference between the "axial" skeleton and the "appendicular" skeleton.

_____

_____

_____

_____

_____

_____

_____

_____

_____

2. What are the five major functions of the skeletal system?

_____

_____

_____

_____

_____

_____

_____

_____

_____

Bone Classification

Instructions: *List one example of a bone in the human body that fits into each of the following categories of bone classification.*

1. long: _____

2. short: _____

3. flat: _____

4. sesamoid: _____

5. irregular: _____

Copyright Goodheart-Willcox Co., Inc.
May not be reproduced or posted to a publicly accessible website.

Labeling

Instructions: *Label the different types of bones in the following image.*

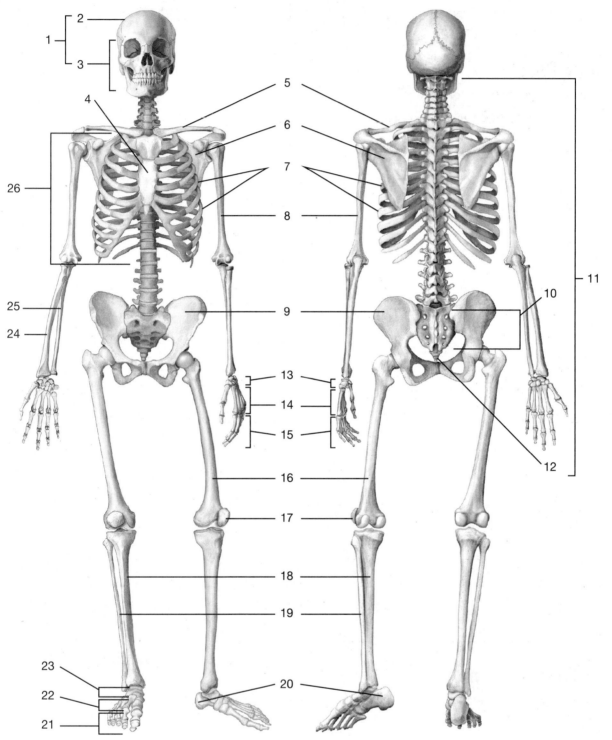

© *Body Scientific International*

1. Item 1:_____

2. Item 2:_____

3. Item 3:_____

4. Item 4:_____

5. Item 5:_____

6. Item 6:_____

7. Item 7:_____

8. Item 8:_____

9. Item 9:_____

10. Item 10:_____

Copyright Goodheart-Willcox Co., Inc.
May not be reproduced or posted to a publicly accessible website.

11. Item 11:_____	19. Item 19:_____
12. Item 12:_____	20. Item 20:_____
13. Item 13:_____	21. Item 21:_____
14. Item 14:_____	22. Item 22:_____
15. Item 15:_____	23. Item 23:_____
16. Item 16:_____	24. Item 24:_____
17. Item 17:_____	25. Item 25:_____
18. Item 18:_____	26. Item 26:_____

Review, Part 2

Instructions: *Answer the following questions.*

1. What is the anatomical term for a bone's growth plate?

   _____

2. Where is the periosteum located?

   _____

3. What does the term *hematopoiesis* mean?

   _____

4. What does the term *articulate* mean?

   _____

Joint Descriptions and Examples

Instructions: *Describe each type of joint and give an example of where each type is found in the body.*

1. Diarthroses:_____

   Example: _____

2. Amphiarthroses: _____

   Example: _____

3. Synarthroses: _____

   Example: _____

Matching

Instructions: *Match each of the following bone-related terms with the correct meaning.*

1. _____ passageway for blood vessels and nerves

2. _____ shallow pit or cavity in or on a bone

3. _____ one of two large processes found on the femur

4. _____ a hollow cavity within a bone

5. _____ areas on bones that extend outward and serve as points of attachment for muscle or tendons

6. _____ a groove or furrow

7. _____ point where cranial bones attach to each other

8. _____ small, round process found on many bones

9. _____ soft spot on an infant's skull

10. _____ large, rough process found on many bones

A. bone processes

B. tubercule

C. trochanter

D. tuberosity

E. fossa

F. foramen

G. sulcus

H. sinus

I. suture

J. fontanel

Copyright Goodheart-Willcox Co., Inc.
May not be reproduced or posted to a publicly accessible website.

Understanding Terms Related to Diseases and Conditions

Disease or Condition Identification

Instructions: *Identify the term that corresponds to each disease or condition described.*

1. inflammation of the sac of fluid that is located near a joint:

   _____

2. a medical condition in which blood uric acid levels are elevated and can cause joint swelling and pain:

   _____

3. joint swelling at the base of the great toe due to inflammation:

   _____

4. luxation:

   _____

5. softening of the cartilage:

   _____

6. rheumatoid arthritis of the spine:

   _____

7. pain in the lower back:

   _____

8. inflammation of the covering that surrounds the bone:

   _____

9. inflammation of the bone and bone marrow:

   _____

10. rickets:

    _____

11. cancer of plasma cells:

    _____

12. partial dislocation of a bone:

    _____

13. clubfoot:

    _____

14. osteitis deformans:

    _____

Copyright Goodheart-Willcox Co., Inc.
May not be reproduced or posted to a publicly accessible website.

Abnormal Curvature Labeling

Instructions: *Label each abnormal curvature of the spine shown in the following images.*

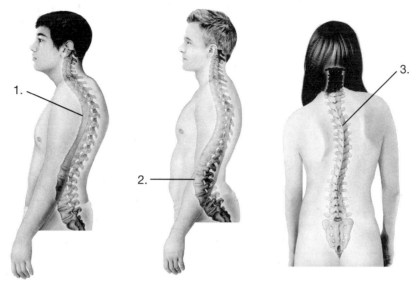

© Body Scientific International

1. Item 1: _____

2. Item 2: _____

3. Item 3: _____

Matching

Instructions: *Match each of the following terms related to fractures with the correct meaning.*

1. _____ a break across the bone at an angle

2. _____ an open fracture

3. _____ a fracture that may be a result of falling onto an outstretched hand

4. _____ a break that is a result of a weakened bone

5. _____ a common fracture seen in sports injuries

6. _____ a fracture primarily seen in children

7. _____ a fracture that splinters or crushes the bone

8. _____ a fracture that may occur because of an excessive impact

A. Colles fracture

B. comminuted fracture

C. greenstick fracture

D. oblique fracture

E. pathologic fracture

F. spiral fracture

G. stress fracture

H. compound fracture

Copyright Goodheart-Willcox Co., Inc.
May not be reproduced or posted to a publicly accessible website.

Activity E   Analyzing Diagnostic- and Treatment-Related Terms

Diagnostic Test Identification

Instructions: *Identify the diagnostic test that would be considered in each of the following situations.*

1. a test that may be used to collect cells that would be used in a stem-cell transplant procedure:

   _____

2. a test that is used to diagnose osteoporosis:

   _____

3. a test that provides more detailed images than a regular X-ray but is not as costly as an MRI:

   _____

Matching

Instructions: *Match each of the following surgical procedures or treatments with the correct meaning.*

1. _____ surgery to repair a fracture that requires the use of plates and screws

2. _____ an artificial limb

3. _____ the application of a pulling force to correct a dislocated shoulder

4. _____ surgical immobilization of a joint

5. _____ a procedure used to remove fluid from within a joint

6. _____ the surgical fusion of vertebrae

7. _____ the surgical removal of a limb

8. _____ the process of rehabilitating a patient so that he or she is able to ambulate after hip replacement surgery

9. _____ the process of transplanting and implanting bone tissue from the pelvic bones to repair a facial bone injury

10. _____ the surgical removal of the sac of fluid that is found near the elbow joint

A. arthrodesis
B. physical therapy
C. bursectomy
D. amputation
E. traction
F. prosthesis
G. spondylosyndesis
H. ORIF
I. arthrocentesis
J. bone grafting

Definitions

Instructions: *Using the word parts on pages 71–73 and Appendix A on pages 473–479 of your textbook, define the following medical terms.*

1. subcostal: _____

2. bradykinesia: _____

3. arthrogram: _____

4. osteoarthritis: _____

5. pedal: _____

Copyright Goodheart-Willcox Co., Inc.
May not be reproduced or posted to a publicly accessible website.

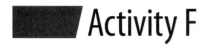 Activity F   Preparing for Your Future
in Healthcare

Word Part Definitions

Instructions: *Define each of the following word parts that are related to healthcare professions.*

1. chir/o: _____

2. neur/o: _____

3. muscul/o: _____

4. ultra-: _____

5. orth/o: _____

6. -ist: _____

7. radi/o: _____

Definitions

Instructions: *Use the Glossary/Index in the text or a dictionary to define the following terms.*

1. manipulation:

   _____

   _____

2. adjunctive:

   _____

   _____

3. acupuncture:

   _____

   _____

4. modification:

   _____

   _____

5. intervention:

   _____

   _____

6. customized:

   _____

   _____

Copyright Goodheart-Willcox Co., Inc.
May not be reproduced or posted to a publicly accessible website.

7. rehabilitation:

_____

_____

8. amputation:

_____

_____

Healthcare Professional Indication

Instructions: *Indicate the appropriate healthcare professional (chiropractor, physical therapist, orthopedic surgeon, prosthetist, radiologic technologist) for each of the following tasks. You will use some of the healthcare professionals more than once.*

1. fabricates artificial limbs:

_____

2. educates people on exercises to improve their mobility:

_____

3. requires a DC degree:

_____

4. requires an MD or a DO degree:

_____

5. takes X-rays of bones:

_____

6. may use acupuncture as a treatment option:

_____

7. may work in a nursing home:

_____

8. is licensed to perform surgery:

_____

9. may practice with an associate's degree:

_____

10. must have a doctor's order before fitting a patient with a prosthesis:

_____

Copyright Goodheart-Willcox Co., Inc.
May not be reproduced or posted to a publicly accessible website.

Chapter 4 Practice Test

Word Part Definition

Instructions: *Using the word parts on pages 71–73 of your textbook, identify the medical term that corresponds to each of the following definitions.*

1. incision into the skull:_____

2. surgical repair of a joint:_____

3. pertaining to below the ribs: _____

4. inflammation of the bones in a joint: _____

5. resembling watery flow: _____

Medical Terms and Definitions

Instructions: *Break down each of the following medical terms into its word parts (prefix, root word, combining vowel, and suffix if used). Then define each term.*

1. subluxation

   Breakdown:_____

   Define:_____

2. osteopenia

   Breakdown:_____

   Define:_____

3. metatarsal

   Breakdown:_____

   Define:_____

4. intracranial

   Breakdown:_____

   Define:_____

5. arthrodesis

   Breakdown:_____

   Define:_____

6. chondroma

   Breakdown:_____

   Define:_____

7. cranioplasty

   Breakdown:_____

   Define:_____

8. myeloma

   Breakdown:_____

   Define:_____

Copyright Goodheart-Willcox Co., Inc.
May not be reproduced or posted to a publicly accessible website.

Bone Labeling

Instructions: *Label each of the following bones as either axial or appendicular depending on the part of the skeletal system in which it is located.*

1. cervical vertebra: _____

2. clavicle: _____

3. frontal bone: _____

4. ribs: _____

5. fibula: _____

6. coccyx: _____

Review, Part 1

Instructions: *Answer the following questions.*

1. Which two minerals are stored inside bones?

_____

2. Which structure attaches bones to muscles?

_____

3. Which term describes the shaft of a long bone?

_____

4. What substance is found at the edge of the growth plate and allows for new bone to form in children?

_____

5. Which term describes the hard, strong, and dense bone that forms the outermost layer of most bones?

_____

6. What is the smallest bone in the body? Where is it located?

_____

Joint Identification

Instructions: *Identify the type of joint shown in each of the following images.*

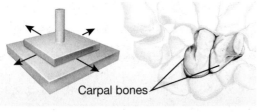

Carpal bones

© Body Scientific International

1. Type of joint: _____

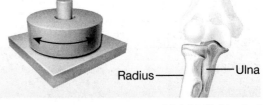

Radius — Ulna

© Body Scientific International

2. Type of joint: _____

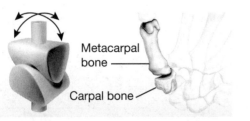

Metacarpal bone

Carpal bone

© Body Scientific International

3. Type of joint: _____

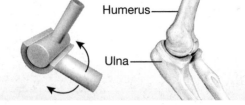

Humerus

Ulna

© Body Scientific International

4. Type of joint: _____

Copyright Goodheart-Willcox Co., Inc.
May not be reproduced or posted to a publicly accessible website.

Name _____

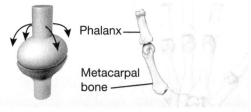

Phalanx —

Metacarpal bone —

© Body Scientific International

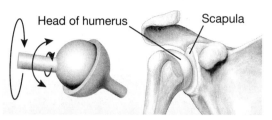

Head of humerus   Scapula

© Body Scientific International

5. Type of joint:_____

6. Type of joint:_____

Disease or Condition Identification

Instructions: *Identify the term that corresponds to each disease or condition described.*

1. inflammation of the sac that contains synovial fluid and is found between bones and muscles:

   _____

2. inflammation of a joint that is caused by elevated levels of uric acid:

   _____

3. a malignant tumor of the connective tissue that affects the bone:

   _____

4. abnormal lateral (side-to-side) curvature of the spine:

   _____

5. the partial dislocation of a joint:

   _____

6. an abnormal depression of the sternum into the chest cavity:

   _____

Fracture Identification

Instructions: *Identify the type of fracture shown in each of the following images.*

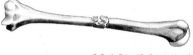

© Body Scientific International

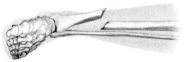

© Body Scientific International

1. Type of fracture: _____

2. Type of fracture: _____

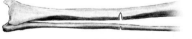

© Body Scientific International

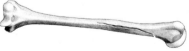

© Body Scientific International

3. Type of fracture: _____

4. Type of fracture: _____

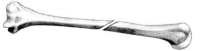

© Body Scientific International

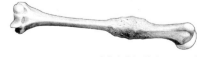

© Body Scientific International

5. Type of fracture: _____

6. Type of fracture: _____

Copyright Goodheart-Willcox Co., Inc.
May not be reproduced or posted to a publicly accessible website.

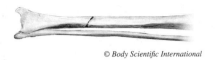

© Body Scientific International

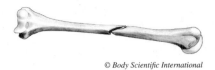

© Body Scientific International

7. Type of fracture: _____   8. Type of fracture: _____

Term Identification

Instructions: *Identify the term that corresponds to each treatment described.*

1. external manipulation to restore a fractured bone to the correct position: _____

2. the incision of a tendon: _____

3. the surgical repair of a bone: _____

4. the surgical removal of a vertebral disk: _____

5. the surgical repair of a joint: _____

6. the surgical removal of a limb: _____

7. an artificial limb: _____

8. the surgical repair of a fracture using hardware, such as pins and plates: _____

Review, Part 2

Instructions: *Answer each question that follows using your knowledge of medical abbreviations.*

1. If a drug is ordered **PRN**, when would a patient take it?

   _____

   _____

2. If an arthroplasty were recommended because of **DJD**, what reason would you give the patient for the surgery?

   _____

   _____

3. If a drug is ordered **PO**, how should the patient take it?

   _____

   _____

4. If the doctor ordered a **BP**, what test would be performed?

   _____

   _____

5. If the medical chart states that the Pt c/o **LBP**, what problem does the patient have?

   _____

   _____

6. If a patient has a compound fracture, and the doctor is scheduling the patient for an **ORIF**, what kind of surgery will the patient be having?

   _____

   _____

7. If a patient's chart states that he or she was treated by the **ATT PHYS** at a hospital, what is that healthcare worker's title?

   _____

   _____

Copyright Goodheart-Willcox Co., Inc.
May not be reproduced or posted to a publicly accessible website.

CHAPTER 5 — The Muscular System

Activity A   Understanding Word Parts

Word Parts Matching, Part 1

Instructions: *Match each of the following word parts with the correct meaning.*

1. _____ breakdown; separation; loosening
2. _____ near; beside; alongside; beyond; abnormal
3. _____ sensation
4. _____ pain
5. _____ slow
6. _____ around
7. _____ paralysis
8. _____ tone; tension
9. _____ process of recording
10. _____ painful; difficult

A. -esthesia
B. -plegia
C. brady-
D. -graphy
E. para-
F. -tonia
G. dys-
H. -dynia
I. -lysis
J. circum-

Word Parts Matching, Part 2

Instructions: *Match each of the following word parts with the correct meaning.*

1. _____ straight; normal
2. _____ smooth
3. _____ muscle
4. _____ sole of the foot
5. _____ coordination; order
6. _____ joint
7. _____ sound
8. _____ movement
9. _____ rod-shaped
10. _____ turn; turning

A. tax/o
B. my/o
C. plant/o
D. son/o
E. orth/o
F. vers/o
G. rhabd/o
H. lei/o
I. kinesi/o
J. articul/o

Copyright Goodheart-Willcox Co., Inc.
May not be reproduced or posted to a publicly accessible website.

Build the Medical Term

Instructions: *Use the combining forms listed on pages 101–102 of your textbook to build the medical term that corresponds to each of the following definitions.*

1. Word part: my/o

   Definition: breakdown of muscle tissue

   Term: _____

2. Word part: son/o

   Definition: process of recording sound

   Term: _____

3. Word part: fasci/o

   Definition: incision into the fibrous band around a muscle

   Term: _____

4. Word part: my/o

   Definition: protrusion of a muscle through a tear

   Term: _____

Medical Terms and Definitions

Instructions: *Break down each of the following medical terms into its word parts (prefix, root word, combining vowel, and suffix if used). Then define each term.*

1. dystrophy

   Breakdown: _____

   Define: _____

2. fibromyalgia

   Breakdown: _____

   Define: _____

3. neuromuscular

   Breakdown: _____

   Define: _____

4. myasthenia

   Breakdown: _____

   Define: _____

5. bradykinesia

   Breakdown: _____

   Define: _____

6. hemiplegic

   Breakdown: _____

   Define: _____

Copyright Goodheart-Willcox Co., Inc.
May not be reproduced or posted to a publicly accessible website.

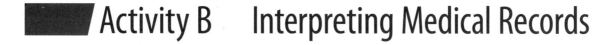

Activity B   Interpreting Medical Records

Term Definitions

Instructions: *Review the case study on page 119 of your textbook. Then use a regular or medical dictionary to define the following terms.*

1. assessment: _____

2. posterior: _____

3. subsided: _____

4. therapeutic: _____

Medical Record Interpretation

Instructions: *Read the following medical record. Identify the meaning of the abbreviations that appear in bold and are listed after the record. Then answer the questions that follow.*

Medical Record

University Rehabilitation Center

Physical Therapy Note

Patient's Name: Timmy Jones

Patient ID Number: 23456

Date of Service: January 12, 20XX

Subjective Data: Pt is a 7 **y/o** male with **hx** of **DMD**. **Dx** was confirmed at age 3 by muscle **Bx** and **NMI**. Recent testing reveals a slight increase in muscular **hypertrophy** of the calves as compared to testing performed approximately 2 years ago. Pt's mother states that pt has increasingly **c/o** difficulty with **amb** and that he "just doesn't like to go outside and play with the neighborhood kids anymore." Pt's mother states that she continues to put his leg splints on at **hs**, but she has noticed that he will take them off during the night. She states that he c/o discomfort when the splints are on. Splints were customized for the Pt approximately 2 years ago. Pt's **PCP** has ordered **PT** evaluation and recommendations for **Tx** modalities.

Objective Data: Pt ambulates to exam table using an adjustable forearm orthopedic crutch, both **L** and **R** sides. Both crutches are extended to the maximum length. Pt's gait is waddling, **dystaxic**, and displays significant toe walking. Pt was able to get onto the exam table using upper extremities and with assistance from therapist.

Physical Exam: Upper extremity **ROM WNL**. Decreased ROM of **bilateral** lower extremities was observed. Also noted a marked decrease in **DTR**, lower extremities bilaterally.

Plan: Develop strengthening exercise program for outpatient PT 3 times a week for 6 weeks. Include **hydrotherapy** and **passive ROM** in Tx plan. Also develop and instruct Pt and mother on home exercise program, including **assisted ROM** to prevent **contractures**. Refer Pt to orthotics for custom fitting of new leg braces and rolling pediatric walker. Refer Pt to home health agency for occupational therapy evaluation and make recommendation for additional adaptive devices.

1. y/o: _____

2. hx: _____

3. DMD: _____

4. Dx: _____

5. Bx: _____

6. NMI: _____

7. c/o: _____

Copyright Goodheart-Willcox Co., Inc.
May not be reproduced or posted to a publicly accessible website.

8. amb: _____

9. hs: _____

10. PCP: _____

11. PT:_____

12. Tx:_____

13. L:_____

14. R: _____

15. ROM: _____

16. WNL: _____

17. DTR: _____

Definitions

Instructions: *Define the following medical terms that appeared in the medical record. Use the word parts lists, the information presented in chapter 5, and the Glossary/Index in the back of your textbook.*

1. hypertrophy: _____

2. dystaxic: _____

3. bilateral: _____

4. hydrotherapy: _____

5. passive ROM: _____

6. assisted ROM:_____

7. contractures: _____

Review

Instructions: *Answer the following questions, referring to the medical record above about Timmy Jones.*

1. Why do you think this patient does not like to walk anymore?

_____

_____

2. Why do you think this patient's leg splints are uncomfortable?

_____

_____

Copyright Goodheart-Willcox Co., Inc.
May not be reproduced or posted to a publicly accessible website.

Name _____

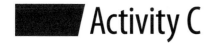 Activity C   Comprehending Anatomy
                    and Physiology Terminology

Review

Instructions: *Answer the following questions.*

1. List the six major functions of the muscular system.

   _____

   _____

   _____

2. What is another name for the skeletal muscle?

   _____

3. What is the name of the structure that holds together skeletal muscle fibers?

   _____

4. What is another name for the smooth muscle?

   _____

5. What is the involuntary movement of smooth muscles?

   _____

6. Where is the cardiac muscle found?

   _____

Word Parts Matching

Instructions: *Match each of the following descriptions with the correct term.*

1. _____ the site at which the muscle is attached to a bone that does not move
   when the muscle contracts

2. _____ the band of fibrous tissue that connects a muscle to a bone

3. _____ the ability of a skeletal muscle to contract

4. _____ the ability of a skeletal muscle to receive and respond to a nerve
   impulse by contracting

5. _____ the involuntary movement of smooth muscles

6. _____ the ability of a muscle to contract without the involvement of nerves

7. _____ the point of attachment of a muscle to a bone that moves during
   muscular contraction

8. _____ the ability of a skeletal muscle to be stretched

9. _____ the ability of skeletal muscle fibers to return to their original resting
   length

10. _____ the band of fibrous tissue that connects a bone to another bone

A. automaticity

B. peristalsis

C. contractility

D. elasticity

E. tendon

F. origin

G. excitability

H. ligament

I. insertion

J. extensibility

Copyright Goodheart-Willcox Co., Inc.
May not be reproduced or posted to a publicly accessible website.

Muscle Labeling

Instructions: *Label the different types of muscles in the following image.*

1. Item 1:

   _____

2. Item 2:

   _____

3. Item 3:

   _____

4. Item 4:

   _____

5. Item 5:

   _____

6. Item 6:

   _____

7. Item 7:

   _____

8. Item 8:

   _____

A. Anterior view   **B. Posterior view**

© *Body Scientific International*

9. Item 9:_____   13. Item 13:_____

10. Item 10:_____   14. Item 14:_____

11. Item 11:_____   15. Item 15:_____

12. Item 12:_____

Muscle Movement

Instructions: *Answer the following questions.*

1. What term describes the movement of the feet when you are standing on "tiptoes" trying to reach something on a high shelf?

   _____

2. What term is used to describe your wrist movement when you reach out your hand to receive money from someone?

   _____

3. What is the position of your knees when you are sitting in a chair with your feet propped up on the table in front of you?

   _____

4. What term describes the movement of your left arm when you turn it with the right hand to look at the back side of your left upper arm?

   _____

Copyright Goodheart-Willcox Co., Inc.
May not be reproduced or posted to a publicly accessible website.

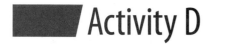 Activity D   Understanding Terms Related
to Diseases and Conditions

Disease Review

Instructions: *Answer the following questions. If you are unsure what a term means, look up the term in the Glossary/Index of your text or use a medical dictionary.*

1. What is a common complication that results from immobilization of or lack of use of a muscle?

   _____

2. Which sex is usually affected by DMD?

   _____

3. After a fracture is healed and the cast has been removed from an arm, the affected arm is generally smaller in size as compared to the unaffected arm. What term describes the condition of the affected arm?

   _____

4. In the case of a stroke, one side of the body is generally affected more than the other side. If there is total paralysis of one side of the body, what term describes this condition?

   _____

5. What term describes the condition that may affect the wrists of people who play video games for excessive amounts of time?

   _____

6. What two terms might you read in a medical chart describing a patient's c/o tenderness in the latissimus dorsi?

   _____

7. What term might an OB/GYN use to describe a benign tumor of the uterus?

   _____

8. Imagine that a day care worker has been sitting on the floor playing with the children for an hour. When she stands up, she experiences an uncomfortable sensation in her feet and lower legs. What term describes this sensation?

   _____

9. Parkinson's disease affects a patient's ability to ambulate. Terms used to describe the posture and gait of a patient with Parkinson's may include bradykinesia, a muscular stiffness called *rigidity*, and shuffling. One of the most prominent signs of Parkinson's is a quaking or shaking of the patient's limbs. What is the term used to describe this sign?

   _____

10. What does the term *hypertrophic cardiomyopathy* mean?

   _____

Copyright Goodheart-Willcox Co., Inc.
May not be reproduced or posted to a publicly accessible website.

Medical Terms and Definitions

Instructions: *Break down each of the following medical terms into its word parts (prefix, root word, combining vowel, and suffix if used). Then define each term.*

1. plantar fasciitis

   Breakdown: _____

   Define: _____

2. rhabdomyoma

   Breakdown: _____

   Define: _____

3. hypothermia

   Breakdown: _____

   Define: _____

4. pathologist

   Breakdown: _____

   Define: _____

5. tendonitis

   Breakdown: _____

   Define: _____

Word Matching

Instructions: *Match each of the following descriptions with the correct term.*

1. _____ pain in a tendon
2. _____ inflammation of a muscle
3. _____ muscle pain
4. _____ loss of muscle tone
5. _____ muscle stiffness
6. _____ softening of a muscle
7. _____ stretching or tearing of a ligament
8. _____ loss of muscle mass due to aging
9. _____ stretching or tearing of a muscle
10. _____ convulsive muscular contraction

A. sarcopenia
B. sprain
C. hypotonia
D. strain
E. myomalacia
F. tenalgia
G. myalgia
H. spasm
I. rigidity
J. myositis

Copyright Goodheart-Willcox Co., Inc.
May not be reproduced or posted to a publicly accessible website.

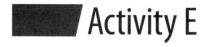 Activity E   Analyzing Diagnostic-
                    and Treatment-Related Terms

Diagnostic Terms

Instructions: *Identify the diagnostic test that would be considered in each of the following situations.*

1. a test to determine the involuntary response of a muscle:

   _____

2. a diagnostic testing method that will visualize soft tissue structures:

   _____

3. a test that measures the electrical activity of a muscle:

   _____

4. a test that uses sound waves to diagnose a leiomyoma:

   _____

Defining Abbreviations

Instructions: *Using the chapter and Appendix B: Medical Abbreviations in the text, define the following abbreviations.*

1. CTS: _____
2. RMS:_____
3. MD:_____
4. ADL:_____
5. CAT: _____
6. DTR: _____
7. NMI: _____

Medical Scenario Treatment

Instructions: *Suppose you are the sports trainer for your school. You have an athlete who has suffered a muscle injury. List the four steps involved in the most common first-aid treatment for muscle injuries. Then, explain how you would teach the athlete what to do to continue the treatment after getting home. Refer to the Medical Record Practice on page 131 of your textbook for additional information.*

1. Step one: _____
2. Step two: _____
3. Step three: _____
4. Step four: _____
5. Home treatment:

   _____

   _____

   _____

Copyright Goodheart-Willcox Co., Inc.
May not be reproduced or posted to a publicly accessible website.

Therapeutic Drug Identification

Instructions: *For each of the following descriptions of a therapeutic drug treatment, indicate the correct term (analgesic, antispasmodic/anticholinergic, narcotic, NSAID) that corresponds with the treatment. You may match more than one term with each description.*

1. treats pain:_____

2. reduces inflammation:_____

3. used to treat smooth muscle spasms: _____

4. aspirin: _____

5. includes OTC medications:_____

6. may cause unconsciousness:_____

7. may be used to treat a fever: _____

Review

Instructions: *Use the table on pages 124–125 and Appendix B of your textbook to answer the following questions.*

1. The orthopedic surgeon has ordered an OTC analgesic to be taken PRN for pain postop arthroscopy. You are going to give the patient instructions for home management. When should you tell the patient to take a pain pill?

   _____

2. A cake decorator has been having symptoms related to CTS. Her PCP has ordered her to wear R wrist splint hs. When will you tell the patient to wear the splint?

   _____

3. You are the nurse on a hospital's orthopedic floor. Your pt is 4 days postop total knee replacement. The surgeon has ordered the intravenous line to be discontinued at 1300 (military time). The patient has been getting pain meds intravenously. The doctor has ordered oral narcotics Q2–3H. At 1430, the patient requests "a pain pill." You quickly fill the order and give the patient the pill. When can you give the patient another pain pill?

   _____

4. You are an ICU nurse taking care of a patient who has been in a car wreck. The patient was given CPR in the ambulance on the way to the hospital. Now, the patient is on a ventilator and not responding to verbal commands. The doctor has ordered you to perform DTR Q8H. Why would the doctor order this test for this patient?

   _____

5. You are the pharmacist and a patient gives you a prescription for the NSAID naproxen 200 mg Q8H. The prescription explains that the patient has a drug allergy to PCN. The patient has been taking an OTC medication for stomach pains. To which medication is this patient allergic?

   _____

6. You are a PFT working at a PT rehabilitation center. You have a new client who had back surgery three months ago and is trying to train for a marathon in six months. What is your job at the rehabilitation center?

   _____

Copyright Goodheart-Willcox Co., Inc.
May not be reproduced or posted to a publicly accessible website.

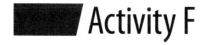 **Activity F   Preparing for Your Future in Healthcare**

Define Word Parts

Instructions: *Define each of the following word parts related to healthcare professionals.*

1. cardi/o: _____

2. myos/o: _____

3. radi/o: _____

4. -metry: _____

Define Terms

Instructions: *Use a dictionary or the Glossary/Index in the back of your textbook to define the following terms.*

1. psychology:

    _____

2. cardiopulmonary resuscitation:

    _____

3. metabolism:

    _____

4. musculoskeletal:

    _____

5. rehabilitation:

    _____

6. diathermy:

    _____

Healthcare Professionals Identification

Instructions: *Identify the appropriate healthcare professional (certified fitness trainer, exercise physiologist, sports medicine physician) that matches each of the following descriptions or tasks. You will use each profession more than once.*

1. performs exercise stress tests:_____

2. requires an MD or DO degree: _____

3. does not require a college degree: _____

4. may work with military pilots who are undergoing endurance training: _____

5. may be the physician for a professional sports team:_____

6. may work in clients' homes to develop personalized exercise programs: _____

7. can prescribe medications: _____

8. may teach yoga and Pilates at a fitness center: _____

9. must have knowledge of the cardiovascular system to effectively develop a training program for clients:

    _____

10. may perform surgery: _____

Copyright Goodheart-Willcox Co., Inc.
May not be reproduced or posted to a publicly accessible website.

Chapter 5 Practice Test

Definitions

Instructions: *Use the word parts on pages 101–102 to build the medical term that corresponds to each of the following definitions.*

1. incision into the fascia: _____

2. the process of bending: _____

3. record of sound: _____

4. muscle in the thigh that has four "heads" or attachments: _____

5. the study of the heart: _____

Medical Terms and Definitions

Instructions: *Break down each of the following medical terms into its word parts (prefix, root word, combining vowel, and suffix if used). Then define each term.*

1. kinesiology

   Breakdown: _____

   Define: _____

2. dorsiflexion

   Breakdown: _____

   Define: _____

3. dystaxia

   Breakdown: _____

   Define: _____

4. myodynia

   Breakdown: _____

   Define: _____

5. tenorrhexis

   Breakdown: _____

   Define: _____

Muscle Identification

Instructions: *Identify which of the following muscles match the correct muscle type (skeletal, smooth, cardiac). You will use each muscle type more than once.*

1. biceps femoris: _____

2. urinary bladder: _____

3. larynx: _____

4. lungs: _____

Copyright Goodheart-Willcox Co., Inc.
May not be reproduced or posted to a publicly accessible website.

5. left ventricle of the heart: _____

6. vertebral column: _____

7. small intestines: _____

8. right atrium of the heart: _____

9. pectoralis major: _____

10. muscles around the lips: _____

Term Identification

Instructions: *Identify each term being described.*

1. The term that describes the ability of the gastrocnemius to be stretched: _____

2. The term that describes the structure surrounding and binding muscle fibers into functional units:

_____

3. The term used to describe the muscle that causes a body part's primary movement:

_____

Directional Movement Identification

Instructions: *Identify the term that corresponds to each directional movement described.*

1. pointing the toes in a straight line away from the body, as when a ballerina stands on the tips of her toes:

_____

2. moving one leg away from the other leg, as in getting up on a horse: _____

3. the rotational movement of the leg when the body is standing erect, the heels of the feet are as close together as possible, and the toes are pointing away from the midline of the body:

_____

4. movement of the wrist when reaching over to pick up a pen from a desk: _____

Matching

Instructions: *Match each of the following muscle functions with the correct muscle.*

1. _____ extends the forearm

2. _____ flexes the thigh, extends the leg

3. _____ flexes the arm and forearm, supinates the hand

4. _____ raises the eyebrows; wrinkles the forehead

5. _____ dorsiflexes and inverts the foot

6. _____ extends the neck; elevates, adducts, and rotates the scapula

7. _____ abducts, flexes, extends, and rotates the arm

8. _____ flexes, adducts, and rotates the arm

9. _____ extends, adducts, and rotates the arm

10. _____ flexes and rotates the thigh; flexes the leg

A. trapezius

B. pectoralis major

C. triceps brachii

D. sartorius

E. rectus femoris

F. latissimus dorsi

G. biceps brachii

H. frontalis

I. deltoid

J. tibialis anterior

Copyright Goodheart-Willcox Co., Inc.
May not be reproduced or posted to a publicly accessible website.

Identifying Terms, Part 1

Instructions: *Identify the term that corresponds to each of the following described diseases or conditions.*

1. total paralysis on one side of the body: _____

2. protrusion of a muscle through a tear: _____

3. loss of muscle mass due to aging: _____

4. inflammation of a muscle: _____

Identifying Terms, Part 2

Instructions: *Identify the term that corresponds to each of the following described medical tests or treatments.*

1. measurement of the degree of motion of a joint in a variety of directions: _____

2. type of physical therapy in which a pool is used to decrease the amount of weight and impact on the joints:

   _____

3. the most common first-aid treatment for muscular injuries:_____

Review Abbreviations

Instructions: *Refer to the medical abbreviations on pages 124–125 of your textbook to answer the following questions.*

1. If a 79 y/o female is reported to have difficulty with amb, what is she having trouble doing?

   _____

2. If the doctor orders a patient to take an OTC analgesic postop, will this patient have to take a written prescription to the pharmacy?

   _____

Copyright Goodheart-Willcox Co., Inc.
May not be reproduced or posted to a publicly accessible website.

The Cardiovascular System

Activity A   Understanding Word Parts

Word Parts Matching, Part 1

Instructions: *Match each of the following word parts with the correct meaning.*

1. _____ in; within
2. _____ above; above normal; excessive
3. _____ pertaining to blood condition
4. _____ slow
5. _____ fast
6. _____ pressure
7. _____ to turn
8. _____ hardening; thickening
9. _____ narrowing; tightening
10. _____ pertaining to

A. -emic
B. brady-
C. -tension
D. hyper-
E. -stenosis
F. tachy-
G. endo-
H. -sclerosis
I. -ous
J. -version

Word Parts Matching, Part 2

Instructions: *Match each of the following word parts with the correct meaning.*

1. _____ lungs
2. _____ narrowing
3. _____ blue
4. _____ clot
5. _____ heart
6. _____ wall; partition
7. _____ stretched; strained
8. _____ to enlarge or expand
9. _____ vessel
10. _____ contraction

A. dilat/o
B. sept/o
C. coron/o
D. pulmon/o
E. systol/o
F. thromb/o
G. angi/o
H. constrict/o
I. cyan/o
J. tens/o

Copyright Goodheart-Willcox Co., Inc.
May not be reproduced or posted to a publicly accessible website.

Build the Medical Term

Instructions: *Use the combining forms listed on pages 135–136 of your textbook to build the medical term that corresponds to each of the following definitions.*

1. Word part: cardi/o

   Definition: inflammation within the heart

   Term: _____

2. Word part: angi/o

   Definition: record or image of a blood vessel

   Term: _____

3. Word part: cardi/o

   Definition: process of recording the electrical activity of the heart

   Term: _____

4. Word part: cardi/o

   Definition: tissue that surrounds the heart

   Term: _____

5. Word part: angi/o

   Definition: surgical repair of a blood vessel

   Term: _____

Medical Terms and Definitions

Instructions: *Break down each of the following medical terms into its word parts (prefix, root word, combining vowel, and suffix if used). Then define each term.*

1. cardiomyopathy

   Breakdown: _____

   Define: _____

2. arteriosclerosis

   Breakdown: _____

   Define: _____

3. thrombophlebitis

   Breakdown: _____

   Define: _____

4. ventriculography

   Breakdown: _____

   Define: _____

5. cardioversion

   Breakdown: _____

   Define: _____

Copyright Goodheart-Willcox Co., Inc.
May not be reproduced or posted to a publicly accessible website.

6. endoarterial

   Breakdown: _____

   Define: _____

7. anticoagulant

   Breakdown: _____

   Define: _____

8. echocardiogram

   Breakdown: _____

   Define: _____

9. cardiologist

   Breakdown: _____

   Define: _____

10. cardiopulmonary

   Breakdown: _____

   Define: _____

Copyright Goodheart-Willcox Co., Inc.
May not be reproduced or posted to a publicly accessible website.

Activity B   Interpreting Medical Records

Instructions: *Read the following medical record. Identify the meaning of the abbreviations that appear in bold and are listed after the record. Then answer the questions that follow.*

Medical Record

<u>County Cardiac Clinic</u>

Patient Name: Harold Smith

Patient ID Number: 87654

Date of Exam: February 14, 20XX

Subjective Data: **Pt** is a 67 **y/o** male **postop CABG** 6 weeks ago. Pt came into the clinic for evaluation for possible cardiac rehab orders. Pt denies any postop complications and states, "I haven't felt this good in years, except for the incision on my leg."

<u>Medications:</u>

Daily: Plavix 300 **mg PO**, Aspirin 325 mg PO, Fish Oil Capsules 1500 mg, Lipitor 50 mg, Lisinopril 25 mg

PRN: Nitrostat Sublingual 0.3 mg, take one when chest pain occurs. May repeat x3 doses. If chest pain continues, contact emergency medical services.

OH: Truck driver for interstate hauling company x45 years.

FH: Father died at age 65 of **CHF**. Mother died at age 82 of **CVA.**

Past Medical **Hx: HTN**; high cholesterol; obesity; smoker x25 years, quit approximately 2 years ago. Denies alcohol or recreational drug use. Admits to occasionally taking "energy" pills when he is on a long haul. Pt states that he normally eats fast food when he is out of town. He does not have a regular exercise program.

History of Present Illness: Pt states that approximately 2 months ago, he was out of town for his job and began having chest tightness, anxiety, sweating, and a feeling of "doom." He went to a minor emergency clinic in the town where he was staying, and was then referred to the **ER** at the local hospital. There he was evaluated for possible **MI**. Cardiac enzymes were elevated, and the **EKG** revealed ST-segment elevation. Pt was prepped for cardiac catheterization. Results of the catheterization showed 2 coronary artery lesions—one on the **LAD** artery and another on the **R** coronary artery. Angioplasty was attempted but was not successful due to the location of the plaque areas in the vessels. Patient requested to be allowed to travel to his hometown for further **tx**. Pt's wife was allowed to transport him back via private vehicle.

Pt was evaluated by his **PCP** and was immediately referred to **CV** department for evaluation of **Dx** of **CAD** and evaluation for possible CABG. Pt underwent this surgery and received 2 bypass grafts. Pt was discharged with skilled home nursing visits for continued monitoring x2 weeks. Pt's recovery period has been uneventful.

Pt states that he is trying to eat a more healthful diet and lower his cholesterol so that he can stop taking Lipitor. Pt states that he has lost almost 30 pounds since surgery, and that he is ready to get doctor's permission to start exercising.

Pt also reports that he has requested that his company transfer him to a local route so he will not be out of town for extended periods of time. He is planning on working for 2–3 more years, when he will be eligible for the maximum retirement benefits from this company. Pt states that he will have someone to help him with deliveries.

<u>Physical Assessment:</u> **wt**: 246 lbs, **ht**: 72 inches

V/S: T: 98.7°, **R**: 14, **P**: 90 **bpm, BP**: 150/92

Midsternal Incision: 31.5 **cm** long. Well healed, some redness at the distal end. Pt states that pain in this area has subsided and only c/o occasional itching. Two incisions on **RLE** related to saphenous vein harvesting, medial proximal incision is 5.2 cm long. Second incision is 25 cm distal to previously mentioned incision. This distal incision is 4.5 cm long. Both incisions are slightly reddened; however, no discharge, warmth, or swelling has been noted. Pt states that these areas have been more worrisome than the incision on his chest.

<u>Plan:</u>

Refer patient to cardiac rehab program for cardiac monitoring during treadmill exercise. Frequency will be 3x week for 4 weeks and re-evaluation.

Recommend that patient not lift anything over 10 pounds.

Refer patient to dietitian for nutritional counseling and weight loss program.

Copyright Goodheart-Willcox Co., Inc.
May not be reproduced or posted to a publicly accessible website.

Name _____

1. Pt: _____

2. y/o: _____

3. postop: _____

4. CABG: _____

5. mg: _____

6. PO: _____

7. PRN: _____

8. OH: _____

9. FH: _____

10. CHF: _____

11. CVA: _____

12. Hx: _____

13. HTN: _____

14. ER: _____

15. MI: _____

16. EKG: _____

17. LAD: _____

18. R: _____

19. tx: _____

20. PCP: _____

21. CV: _____

22. Dx: _____

23. CAD: _____

24. wt: _____

25. ht: _____

26. V/S: _____

27. T: _____

28. R: _____

29. P: _____

30. bpm: _____

31. BP: _____

32. cm: _____

33. RLE: _____

34. What is the reason for the incision on this patient's leg?

_____

_____

35. What are some reasons that contribute to this patient's risk for developing heart problems?

_____

_____

Copyright Goodheart-Willcox Co., Inc.
May not be reproduced or posted to a publicly accessible website.

⬛◣ Activity C   Comprehending Anatomy and Physiology Terminology

Review

Instructions: *Answer the following questions.*

1. What is the primary purpose of the cardiovascular system?

_____

_____

2. Which terms describe the three layers of the heart?

_____

3. Which term describes the upper chambers of the heart?

_____

4. Which term describes the bottom chambers of the heart?

_____

5. What two gases does the blood distribute to the cells and lungs?

_____

6. What are the two major components of blood?

_____

Terms Matching

Instructions: *Match each of the following anatomical terms with the correct function or description.*

1. _____ valve with three flaps located in the aorta

2. _____ carries oxygen-poor blood to the heart from the upper part of the body

3. _____ general term that describes any blood vessel that carries oxygen-rich blood away from the heart

4. _____ the site where oxygen is delivered to the body's tissues and cells

5. _____ valve with three flaps located in the pulmonary artery

6. _____ general term that describes any blood vessel that carries oxygen-poor blood back toward the heart from the body

7. _____ located between the right atrium and the right ventricle

8. _____ blood vessel that carries blood away from the right ventricle into the pulmonary circulation system

9. _____ the largest artery in the body, which carries oxygen-rich blood away from the heart into the systemic circulation system

10. _____ blood vessel that carries blood from the lungs to the left atrium of the heart

A. capillaries

B. veins

C. arteries

D. aorta

E. tricuspid valve

F. superior vena cava

G. pulmonary veins

H. aortic semilunar valve

I. pulmonary arteries

J. pulmonary semilunar valve

Copyright Goodheart-Willcox Co., Inc.
May not be reproduced or posted to a publicly accessible website.

Artery Identification

Instructions: *Label the missing arteries in the following image.*

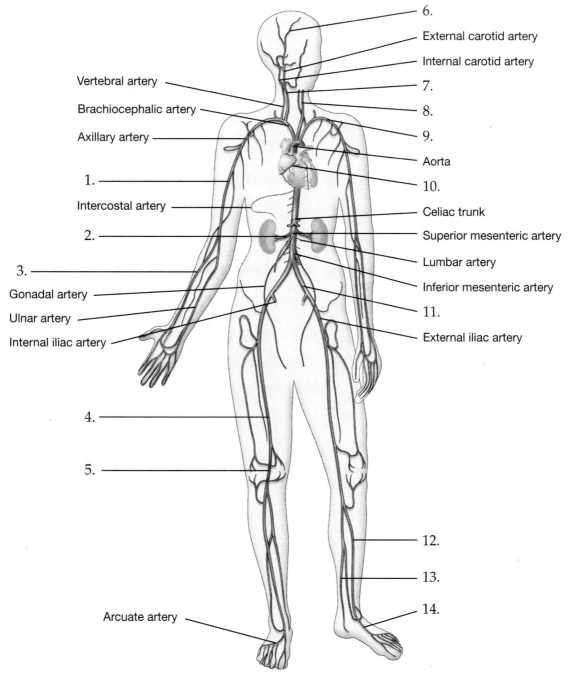

6.

External carotid artery

Internal carotid artery

Vertebral artery

7.

Brachiocephalic artery

8.

Axillary artery

9.

1.

Aorta

Intercostal artery

10.

Celiac trunk

2.

Superior mesenteric artery

3.

Lumbar artery

Gonadal artery

Inferior mesenteric artery

Ulnar artery

11.

Internal iliac artery

External iliac artery

4.

5.

Arcuate artery

12.

13.

14.

© *Body Scientific International*

1. Item 1:_____

2. Item 2:_____

3. Item 3:_____

4. Item 4:_____

5. Item 5:_____

6. Item 6:_____

7. Item 7:_____

8. Item 8:_____

9. Item 9:_____

10. Item 10:_____

11. Item 11:_____

12. Item 12:_____

13. Item 13:_____

14. Item 14:_____

Copyright Goodheart-Willcox Co., Inc.
May not be reproduced or posted to a publicly accessible website.

Activity D   Understanding Terms Related to Diseases and Conditions

Nurse Practitioner Medical Scenarios

Instructions: *Read the following scenarios and answer the question in each one. For the following scenarios, suppose you are a nurse practitioner in a cardiology office.*

1. The first patient you see has a pulse rate of 42 bpm. You know that a normal rate is between 60 and 100 bpm. How would you document this patient's heart rate?

   _____

2. The next patient has a resting heart rate of 125. How would you document this heart rate?

   _____

3. The next patient was booked as an urgent appointment. She has been complaining of pressure in her chest since 4:00 a.m. This patient was evaluated in the ER at 6:00 a.m. and was referred to your office. Which term would you use to document this patient's complaints of chest pain?

   _____

4. You schedule the previous patient for cardiac catheterization to determine if she has arteriosclerosis. She asks you to tell her what *arteriosclerosis* means. How do you describe this condition to her?

   _____

   _____

   _____

5. On your schedule, you see that your next patient has chronic CHF. What are some questions you will ask him to determine whether his condition is worsening?

   _____

   _____

6. When you examine the patient with chronic CHF, you tell him that he has more cyanosis than before. He asks you to explain what you mean. What do you tell him?

   _____

   _____

   _____

7. This patient's blood pressure is 90/45. You know that a normal blood pressure range is 90–140/60–90. Which condition would you document for this patient?

   _____

8. The medical assistant has already checked your next patient's blood pressure and recorded it as 170/96. Which condition would you document for this patient?

   _____

Copyright Goodheart-Willcox Co., Inc.
May not be reproduced or posted to a publicly accessible website.

9. After your lunch break, the first patient you see has a new diagnosis of mitral valve prolapse. She asks you to explain this condition. How will you explain mitral valve prolapse?

_____

_____

_____

10. When you perform your examination on this patient with your stethoscope, you hear an abnormal sound. You know this sound occurs because the mitral valve is not closing completely. How would you document this in the medical record?

_____

11. Your last patient of the afternoon is a healthy, elderly patient who walks 3–5 miles every day. However, today he tells you that, in the past two weeks, he has not been able to walk more than half of a mile because he experiences pains in his calf. When he stops to rest, the pain goes away, but it comes back as soon as he starts walking again. What condition do you think this patient is experiencing?

_____

12. Which term will you use to describe your elderly patient's intermittent pain?

_____

13. Imagine that you are a nurse in a busy ER. A gunshot victim is transported to your facility via ambulance. There is a large amount of blood on the gurney. The Hbg test in the ER shows that the pt's hemoglobin level is at 8 g/dL. You recall that normal hemoglobin values for men are 13.5 to 17.5 g/dL. You notify the attending ER doctor of the patient's hemoglobin levels. The doctor tells you to perform a test to check for blood-type compatibility on this patient. Which test will you identify on the lab request slip?

_____

14. The lab result on the test from the previous question shows that the patient has a blood type of AB positive. The ER doctor orders a procedure in which blood will be administered to the pt. You fill out the request slip for the blood bank. Which procedure will you order for this patient?

_____

Charge Nurse Medical Scenarios

Instructions: *For the following scenarios, suppose you are the charge nurse in the cardiac care wing of the hospital. You are reviewing the patient load so that you can assign patients to your incoming nurses for the evening shift.*

1. In room 1421, you have Mr. Johnson, a 70 y/o male who was transferred to your floor from the Coronary Intensive Care Unit after having an angioplasty performed the day before. He has a diagnosis of CAD. You are going to instruct your nurse to teach this patient about CAD. How do you expect your nurse to describe this condition?

_____

_____

_____

2. In room 1412, you have Mrs. Rogers, who is 3 days postop for the repair of an abdominal aortic aneurysm. You are going to assign this patient to a nurse who just graduated from nursing school. How will you explain to this nurse the reason for the patient's surgery?

_____

_____

Copyright Goodheart-Willcox Co., Inc.
May not be reproduced or posted to a publicly accessible website.

3. In room 1423, you have Mrs. Smith, who was admitted from the ER earlier today with a blood clot in the vein of her lower left leg. The vein is inflamed, and the patient complains of pain in the extremity. What is this patient's likely diagnosis?

_____

4. Mr. Taylor is a 45 y/o male in room 1418 who is currently receiving intravenous antibiotic therapy to treat a bacterial infection that has caused inflammation of the inner layer of his heart. How would you document this patient's condition?

_____

5. You check the heart monitors of the patients on your floor and you notice that Mr. Jones in room 1415 has rapid, spontaneous contractions of the atria. You contact Mr. Jones' cardiologist with this information. How does the cardiologist describe Mr. Jones' condition?

_____

_____

_____

6. Later in the shift, you are visiting with the recent nursing school graduate, who is preparing to take the state board exam for his nursing license. He tells you that he has noticed his heart sometimes seems to have an irregular rhythm. You put an extra heart monitor on him and notice that he does have an extra, abnormal heartbeat that occasionally disrupts the regular ventricular rhythm of his heart. What condition does this nurse have?

_____

7. You have a nurse who tells you that she is going to be off work for the next few days to have her varicose veins removed. How can you verify that she has this condition?

_____

_____

_____

8. When you check on Mr. Johnson in room 1421, he tells you that the healthcare workers in the cardiac catheterization lab kept referring to his "MI." Since Mr. Johnson received sedation prior to the procedure, he could not remember what the healthcare workers told him about this condition. How do you explain to him what "MI" means?

_____

_____

_____

9. The 58 y/o male patient was referred to oncology by his dermatologist because his test came back as malignant melanoma. You are to draw blood and send it to the lab for a series of tests. One of the tests will check for the ability of the patient's blood to clot. What is the name of this test?

_____

Copyright Goodheart-Willcox Co., Inc.
May not be reproduced or posted to a publicly accessible website.

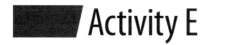 **Activity E   Analyzing Diagnostic-**
and Treatment-Related Terms

Terms Matching

Instructions: *Match each of the following terms with the correct meaning.*

1. _____ procedure in which a radioactive substance is injected into a vein near the end of a stress test to determine the sizes of the heart chambers, how well the heart is pumping blood, and if there is any tissue damage in the heart

2. _____ test that uses a radioactive "tracer" to look for disease or poor blood flow in the heart

3. _____ an instrument used to determine blood pressure

4. _____ the process of listening to the internal body sounds

5. _____ test that uses a "tracer" to measure the volume of blood that is pumped by the ventricles

6. _____ tool that is used to listen to internal body sounds

7. _____ the procedure in which blood flow is measured using high-frequency sound waves

8. _____ test in which a tiny plastic tube is inserted into a blood vessel, usually the femoral artery, to diagnose heart diseases or abnormalities

9. _____ the measurement of a patient's cardiovascular health during exercise, usually on a treadmill

10. _____ term for the pressure exerted by the blood against the walls of a blood vessel

A. auscultation
B. blood pressure
C. nuclear ventriculography
D. exercise stress test
E. nuclear thallium stress test
F. stethoscope
G. Doppler ultrasound
H. cardiac catheterization
I. PET scan
J. sphygmomanometer

Term Identification

Instructions: *Identify the term that corresponds to each treatment method described below.*

1. electrical device that is implanted in the chest to control abnormal cardiac rhythms:

_____

2. electrical device that is implanted in the chest to specifically control atrial or ventricular fibrillation:

_____

3. wire mesh tube that is inserted into an artery to prevent the artery from becoming blocked:

_____

4. procedure that sends controlled electrical shocks to the heart in an effort to restore normal cardiac rhythm:

_____

5. passageway that is established surgically, allowing blood to travel from the aorta to a branch of the coronary artery at a point beyond an obstruction:

_____

Copyright Goodheart-Willcox Co., Inc.
May not be reproduced or posted to a publicly accessible website.

Matching

Instructions: *Match each of the following cardiac medications with the effect it has on the body.*

1. _____ helps reduce the amount of water in the body

2. _____ dilates the arteries and reduces blood pressure

3. _____ general term for any medication that is used to reduce blood pressure

4. _____ prevents the body from making angiotensin II

5. _____ reduces lipid levels in the blood

6. _____ prevents or reduces angina

7. _____ used to treat several conditions, including angina, hypertension, irregular heart rhythms, migraines, panic attacks, and tremors

8. _____ constricts or narrows blood vessels

9. _____ prevents or reduces irregular rhythms of the heart

10. _____ helps dissolve blood clots

A. thrombolytic

B. beta blocker

C. antianginal

D. diuretic

E. hypolipidemic

F. vasoconstrictor

G. antihypertensive

H. antiarrhythmic

I. ACE inhibitor

J. calcium channel blocker

Copyright Goodheart-Willcox Co., Inc.
May not be reproduced or posted to a publicly accessible website.

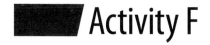 # Activity F   Preparing for Your Future in Healthcare

Definitions

Instructions: *Refer to the description of healthcare professionals on page 167 in your textbook. Then define the following terms. You may use the information in your textbook, a regular or medical dictionary, the Glossary/Index in the back of your textbook, and your own words to define the terms.*

1. electrocardiogram: _____

_____

2. sonography: _____

_____

3. cardiac catheterization: _____

_____

4. Holter monitor: _____

_____

5. stress test: _____

_____

6. cardioversion: _____

_____

7. arrhythmia: _____

_____

8. fibrillation: _____

_____

9. defibrillation: _____

_____

10. nuclear thallium stress test: _____

_____

Matching

Instructions: *Match the appropriate healthcare professional (cardiologist, cardiovascular technician, telemetry nurse) with each of the following descriptions or tasks. You will use each profession more than once.*

1. requires a medical degree: _____

2. may supervise LPNs and CNAs: _____

3. may work with physicians in a cardiac catheterization lab: _____

4. can order heart testing for patients: _____

5. monitors patient's heart rhythms while patient is in the hospital: _____

Copyright Goodheart-Willcox Co., Inc.
May not be reproduced or posted to a publicly accessible website.

Chapter 6 Practice Test

Definitions

Instructions: *Using the word parts on pages 135–136 of your textbook, define the following medical terms.*

1. bradycardia:

   _____

   _____

2. cardiomyopathy:

   _____

   _____

3. thrombophlebitis:

   _____

   _____

4. angioplasty:

   _____

   _____

5. electrocardiologist:

   _____

   _____

6. hemoglobin:

   _____

   _____

Build the Medical Term

Instructions: *Use the following combining forms and suffixes listed on pages 135–136 of your textbook to build the medical term that corresponds to each of the following definitions.*

1. Word part: angi/o

   Definition: narrowing or tightening of a blood vessel

   Term: _____

2. Word part: -ary

   Definition: pertaining to the lungs

   Term: _____

3. Word part: -ary

   Definition: pertaining to the heart and lungs

   Term: _____

Copyright Goodheart-Willcox Co., Inc.
May not be reproduced or posted to a publicly accessible website.

4. Word part: -al

   Definition: pertaining to the wall between the chambers of the heart

   Term: _____

5. Word part: -ation

   Definition: condition of excessive clotting

   Term: _____

Medical Terms and Definitions

Instructions: *Break down each of the following medical terms into its words parts (prefix, root word, combining vowel, and suffix if used). Then define each term.*

1. septoplasty

   Breakdown: _____

   Define: _____

2. hypotrophy

   Breakdown: _____

   Define: _____

3. coagulopathy

   Breakdown: _____

   Define: _____

4. perivascular

   Breakdown: _____

   Define: _____

5. transvascular

   Breakdown: _____

   Define: _____

Review

Instructions: *Answer the following questions.*

1. Which term describes the sac that surrounds the heart?

   _____

2. Which term is used to identify the valve between the left atrium and the left ventricle?

   _____

3. Which term describes the sound heard through auscultation when the atrioventricular valves close?

   _____

4. Which term describes the structure in the nodal system where an electrical impulse terminates?

   _____

5. What is considered a normal systolic blood pressure range?

   _____

Copyright Goodheart-Willcox Co., Inc.
May not be reproduced or posted to a publicly accessible website.

6. Where in the body would you find the popliteal artery?

   _____

7. Which term describes the buildup of plaque in arteries that can lead to tissue damage in the heart?

   _____

8. What is the term for a mass of plaque that travels through the bloodstream and can cause a blood vessel to become occluded, or obstructed?

   _____

9. Which tool is used to measure blood pressure?

   _____

10. Where on the body is a person's pulse detected?

    _____

11. Which surgical procedure involves removing plaque from the lining of an artery?

    _____

12. Which term describes the minimally invasive procedure in which a coronary artery is opened to allow better blood flow to the heart muscle?

    _____

13. Which classification of drugs will help reduce the lipid (fat) levels in the blood?

    _____

14. Which classification of drugs may be used to dissolve a thrombus?

    _____

15. Which classification of drugs stimulates the widening of a blood vessel to maintain proper blood flow?

    _____

16. Which term describes the condition caused by a lack of vitamin B_{12}?

    _____

Copyright Goodheart-Willcox Co., Inc.
May not be reproduced or posted to a publicly accessible website.

CHAPTER 7 — The Lymphatic and Immune Systems

Activity A   Understanding Word Parts

Word Parts Matching, Part 1

Instructions: *Match each of the following word parts with the correct meaning.*

1. _____ not; without
2. _____ enlargement
3. _____ change; beyond
4. _____ love; attraction for
5. _____ breakdown; separation; loosening
6. _____ across
7. _____ pertaining to blood condition
8. _____ formation
9. _____ many
10. _____ eat; swallow

A. poly-
B. -lysis
C. -emic
D. -phage
E. meta-
F. trans-
G. -megaly
H. an-
I. -philia
J. -poiesis

Word Parts Matching, Part 2

Instructions: *Match each of the following word parts with the correct meaning.*

1. _____ red
2. _____ blood
3. _____ poison
4. _____ vein
5. _____ lymphatic vessel
6. _____ nucleus
7. _____ clot
8. _____ tonsils
9. _____ white
10. _____ physician; treatment

A. leuk/o
B. phleb/o
C. tox/o
D. hemat/o
E. lymphangi/o
F. iatr/o
G. erythr/o
H. tonsil/o
I. thromb/o
J. kary/o

Copyright Goodheart-Willcox Co., Inc.
May not be reproduced or posted to a publicly accessible website.

Build the Medical Term

Instructions: *Use the combining forms and suffixes listed on pages 173–175 of your textbook to build the medical term that corresponds to each of the following definitions.*

1. Word part: hemat/o

   Definition: formation of blood cells

   Term: _____

2. Word part: -logy

   Definition: study of shape or form

   Term: _____

3. Word part: hem/o

   Definition: bursting forth of blood

   Term: _____

4. Word part: hem/o

   Definition: stop the flow of blood

   Term: _____

5. Word part: -osis

   Definition: abnormal condition of a clot

   Term: _____

Medical Terms and Definitions

Instructions: *Break down each of the following medical terms into its word parts (prefix, root word, combining vowel, and suffix if used). Then define each term.*

1. megakaryocyte

   Breakdown: _____

   Define: _____

2. phlebotomy

   Breakdown: _____

   Define: _____

3. thrombocytopenia

   Breakdown: _____

   Define: _____

4. metamorphosis

   Breakdown: _____

   Define: _____

5. serology

   Breakdown: _____

   Define: _____

Copyright Goodheart-Willcox Co., Inc.
May not be reproduced or posted to a publicly accessible website.

6. neoplasm

   Breakdown: _____

   Define: _____

7. immunosuppression

   Breakdown: _____

   Define: _____

8. lymphoma

   Breakdown: _____

   Define: _____

9. hematocrit

   Breakdown: _____

   Define: _____

10. thrombolytic

   Breakdown: _____

   Define: _____

Copyright Goodheart-Willcox Co., Inc.
May not be reproduced or posted to a publicly accessible website.

Activity B   Interpreting Medical Records

Medical Record Interpretation

Instructions: *Read the following medical record. Identify the meaning of the abbreviations that appear in bold and are listed after the record. Then answer the questions that follow.*

Medical Record

PCP Services of Your Town USA

Patient Name: Sue Smith

Patient ID Number: 56789

Date of Exam: August 28, 20XX

Subjective Data: **Pt** is a 58 **y/o** female with **c/o** increased fatigue x 3 weeks. Pt also reports that during her most recent **BSE**, she noted several swollen areas in her **R** and **L** armpit areas. Pt c/o slight tenderness. Denies redness or irritation on either side. Pt reports that her last mammography showed **bilateral** benign **fibrocystic breast changes.**

Medications: Multivitamins, fish oil capsules, calcium supplements, 81 **mg** aspirin every morning. Pt also takes **OTC NSAID PRN** for **LBP** and OTC omeprazole PRN for occasional **GERD** symptoms. Pt reports allergy to **PCN**.

SH: NS, has occasional glass of wine with dinner, denies recreational drug use.

OH: Recently retired school counselor

FH: Mother died at age 72 of breast cancer. Father died at age 76 of non-Hodgkins lymphoma. Pt has one younger sister who is reportedly in good health. Pt has a twin sister who had a mastectomy approximately 3 years ago. Pt had older brother who died at age 54 of a **MI**.

Objective Data: Review of systems:

HEENT: Denies **HA**, dizziness. Reports **VA WNL**. No **lymphadenomegaly** noted in neck area.

Respiratory: Denies **SOB**. Lungs clear to auscultation.

CV: Denies chest pain, palpitations.

GI: Denies **dyspepsia**, **N/V**. Occasional c/o constipation, approximately twice a month.

GU: Denies dysuria or hematuria.

Neurological: Denies **syncope**, seizure, weakness, or **paresthesia. PERRLA**

Physical Assessment: **wt**: 165 pounds, **ht**: 64 inches

V/S: T: 98.6°, **R**: 14, **P**: 72, **BP**: 142/82

Axillary (armpit) area examined. R side: 2 swollen areas noted, consistent with lymph nodes. One measured 2.0 **cm** x 1.8 cm and medial to this one measured 1.2 cm x 1.2 cm. On the L axillary area, one swollen area noted. This area is more medial than the two on the R side. The lesion on the L side measures 2.5 cm x 2.3 cm. Pt verbalized slight discomfort upon palpation of these areas.

Plan:

Lab: **CBC**, **Hct**, **Hgb**, **WBC** with **diff**, **T3**, **T4**, **TSH**.

X-ray: **CXR**, mammogram, **CT** of bilateral axillary area to **R/O** lymphoma, breast cancer.

1. PCP: _____

2. Pt: _____

3. y/o: _____

4. c/o: _____

5. BSE: _____

6. R: _____

7. L: _____

8. mg: _____

9. OTC: _____

10. NSAID: _____

11. PRN: _____

12. LBP: _____

Copyright Goodheart-Willcox Co., Inc.
May not be reproduced or posted to a publicly accessible website.

13. GERD: _____ 31. V/S: _____

14. PCN: _____ 32. T: _____

15. SH: _____ 33. R: _____

16. NS: _____ 34. P: _____

17. OH: _____ 35. BP: _____

18. MI: _____ 36. cm: _____

19. HEENT: _____ 37. lab: _____

20. HA: _____ 38. CBC: _____

21. VA: _____ 39. Hct: _____

22. WNL: _____ 40. Hgb: _____

23. SOB: _____ 41. WBC: _____

24. CV: _____ 42. diff: _____

25. GI: _____ 43. T_3: _____

26. N/V: _____ 44. T_4: _____

27. GU: _____ 45. TSH: _____

28. PERRLA: _____ 46. CXR: _____

29. wt: _____ 47. CT: _____

30. ht: _____ 48. R/O: _____

Medical Record Definitions

Instructions: *Define the following terms that appeared in the medical record and then answer the question below. You may need to use a medical dictionary as well as the glossary in the text.*

1. bilateral: _____

2. fibrocystic breast changes: _____

3. lymphadenomegaly: _____

4. dyspepsia: _____

5. syncope: _____

6. paresthesia: _____

7. Why do you think the healthcare provider suspected a possible diagnosis of cancer for this patient?

_____

_____

_____

Copyright Goodheart-Willcox Co., Inc.
May not be reproduced or posted to a publicly accessible website.

Activity C   Comprehending Anatomy and Physiology Terminology

Review

Instructions: *Answer the following questions.*

1. Name the two main fluids present in the body.

   _____

2. What do lymph nodes filter?

   _____

3. What is the largest lymphatic organ in the body?

   _____

Define Word Parts

Instructions: *Using the word parts on pages 173–175 of your textbook, define the following medical terms.*

1. erythrocyte: _____

2. thrombocyte: _____

3. leukocyte: _____

4. polymorphonuclear: _____

5. hemolysis: _____

6. phagocytosis: _____

Matching: Cell Types

Instructions: *Match each of the following cell types with the correct meaning.*

1. _____ contains histamine and heparin; also involved in inflammatory reactions

2. _____ detects and destroys foreign cells

3. _____ targets pathogenic cells by recognizing sugars present on them

4. _____ aids in the process of blood clotting; also called a *blood platelet*

5. _____ composed of proteins that act as antibodies

6. _____ attaches to antigens and attacks them

7. _____ causes inflammation during an allergic reaction

A. eosinophil
B. basophil
C. natural killer cell
D. gamma globulin
E. lymphocyte
F. cytotoxic cell
G. thrombocyte

Copyright Goodheart-Willcox Co., Inc.
May not be reproduced or posted to a publicly accessible website.

Identification

Instructions: *Label the structures of the lymphatic system in the following image.*

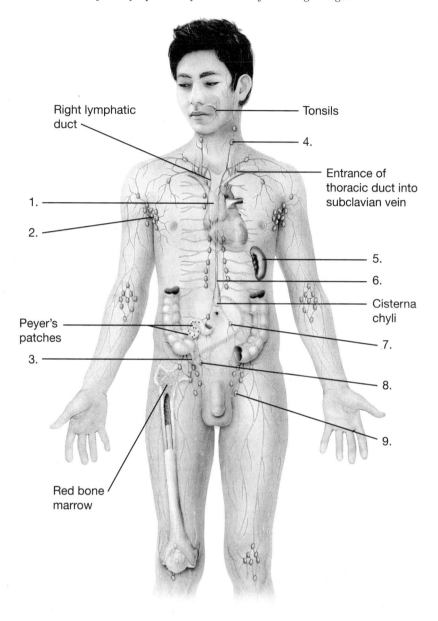

Right lymphatic duct

Tonsils

4.

Entrance of thoracic duct into subclavian vein

1.

2.

5.

6.

Cisterna chyli

7.

Peyer's patches

3.

8.

9.

Red bone marrow

© Body Scientific International

1. Item 1: _____

2. Item 2: _____

3. Item 3: _____

4. Item 4: _____

5. Item 5: _____

6. Item 6: _____

7. Item 7: _____

8. Item 8: _____

9. Item 9: _____

Copyright Goodheart-Willcox Co., Inc.
May not be reproduced or posted to a publicly accessible website.

Matching: B Cells

Instructions: *Match each of the following classes of B cells with the correct meaning.*

1. _____ attached to surface of B cells
2. _____ acts as a powerful clotting agent
3. _____ found in breast milk
4. _____ found in the respiratory tract
5. _____ makes up 75% of all immunoglobulins

A. Immunoglobulin A
B. Immunoglobulin D
C. Immunoglobulin E
D. Immunoglobulin G
E. Immunoglobulin M

Copyright Goodheart-Willcox Co., Inc.
May not be reproduced or posted to a publicly accessible website.

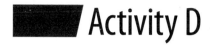 ## Activity D   Understanding Terms Related to Diseases and Conditions

Matching

Instructions: *Match each of the following lymphatic conditions with the correct meaning.*

1. _____ enlargement of the spleen

2. _____ swelling

3. _____ disorder in which one or more parts of the immune system are deficient or missing

4. _____ infection-fighting chemicals released into the bloodstream that trigger inflammation throughout the body

5. _____ hypersensitive reaction by the body to an allergen

6. _____ severe, potentially life-threating allergic reaction

7. _____ malignant cancer of the lymph nodes and lymphatic tissue

8. _____ acute, infectious illness

9. _____ suppression of the immune response caused by HIV

10. _____ cancer of the bone marrow that results in increased amount of WBCs

A. splenomegaly
B. acquired immunodeficiency syndrome (AIDS)
C. lymphoma
D. immunodeficiency disorder
E. leukemia
F. anaphylaxis
G. edema
H. allergy
I. sepsis
J. mononucleosis (mono)

Identification

Instructions: *Identify the term that corresponds to each of the classifications of diseases and conditions described below.*

1. disease in which the body attacks itself, such as SLE and RA:

   _____

2. an infection that appears after someone has been in the hospital:

   _____

3. a condition with no known cause:

   _____

4. an allergy:

   _____

5. a condition that is present at birth:

   _____

6. a sudden outbreak of a contagious disease that affects a large group of people:

   _____

7. a new abnormal growth:

   _____

8. an infection caused by a microorganism that generally does not cause an infection unless someone's immune system has been weakened:

   _____

9. a condition or disease that has no cure and will result in death:

   _____

10. the time period after someone has been sick but is improving:

   _____

Copyright Goodheart-Willcox Co., Inc.
May not be reproduced or posted to a publicly accessible website.

Activity E   Analyzing Diagnostic-
and Treatment-Related Terms

Instructions: *Read the following scenarios and determine which test or medication would be used in each case.*

1. Suppose you are the medical assistant at a primary care clinic. Your first patient of the day is Angela, a 16 y/o who is on her high school's swim team. She has been c/o being tired and unable to practice as long as she used to without resting. She has been experiencing heavy bleeding during her periods for the past 6 months. Her PCP is concerned that she may have anemia. The PCP has ordered a routine lab test to determine the number of RBCs, WBC diff, and platelets that Angela has in her system. You are going to fill out the lab request slip. Which test will you request for Angela?

   _____

2. Suppose you are the receptionist for an immunologist. Your physician hands you a lab request slip for a test to determine the levels of immunoglobulins present in a patient's blood. You are to verify that all the information is correct before you submit the request. What is the name of this test?

   _____

3. Next, the doctor hands you a chart for a patient for whom he is recommending allergy shots to treat severe allergies. You are to make sure the insurance company will cover this procedure. What is the name of the procedure for which you will request preauthorization from the insurance company?

   _____

4. The next patient who comes into the clinic has severe allergies and needs treatment because he is going out of town for a business meeting next week. The physician gives this patient an injection of Kenalog, a hormone-like drug that will decrease inflammation. You are completing the electronic chart to send to the patient's insurance company. What term will you use to describe the drug's classification?

   _____

5. The next patient comes in c/o severe dysuria and hematuria. She states that she has had a fever between 100° and 102° for the past 2 days. She has taken OTC antipyretic medications such as acetaminophen, but the fever has not gone down. You suspect she has a UTI. You order a UA, which confirms your diagnosis. You order Bactrim, a drug that fights bacterial infections. What is this drug's classification?

   _____

6. Your next patient is a 17 y/o male who is the running back on his football team. He has a severe case of athlete's foot. He has been trying OTC products with no improvement in his symptoms of itching and burning. You give him a prescription for Clioquinol to treat his fungal infection. What is this drug's classification?

   _____

7. In the next exam room, you have a 28 y/o female who states that her 2 y/o daughter came home today with symptoms of the flu. Your patient is a busy executive, and she states, "I don't have time to get the flu." She explains that she had the flu vaccine about 3 months ago. You give her a prescription for Tamiflu to prevent and treat the viral infection of influenza. What is this drug's classification?

   _____

8. Suppose you are the oncology nurse at a cancer treatment center. The first patient of the day is a 58 y/o male. He recently had a procedure in which his dermatologist made an incision into a suspicious mole on his right posterior shoulder, removing a piece of the tissue and sending it to the pathology lab for examination. The patient wants to know the name of the procedure he received. What do you tell him?

   _____

Copyright Goodheart-Willcox Co., Inc.
May not be reproduced or posted to a publicly accessible website.

9. The next patient you see in your office is a 55 y/o female who had a mastectomy due to breast cancer. She has undergone radiation therapy, and she is now ready to start the drug therapy of Methotrexate, which is used to prevent the growth of a neoplasm. What is this drug's classification?

_____

10. The next patient is a 24 y/o male with a diagnosis of non-Hodgkin's lymphoma. You are to prepare him for a test in which a small amount of his bone marrow will be removed by a needle for evaluation. What is the name of this test?

_____

11. In the next exam room, you have a 25 y/o female who has been receiving treatment for lymphoma for the past year. She is in the room with her 28 y/o sister, who has undergone testing and been approved as a perfect match for bone marrow donation. Your patient is excited and ready to have the procedure in which some of her sister's bone marrow will be injected into her body. Which term describes this procedure?

_____

Activity F Preparing for Your Future in Healthcare

Definitions

Instructions: *Using the word parts on pages 173–175 of your textbook, determine the area in which each of the following healthcare professionals specializes.*

1. hematologist:

_____

2. pathologist:

_____

3. morphologist:

_____

4. virologist:

_____

5. cytologist:

_____

6. serologist:

_____

Defining Medical Terms

Instructions: *Define the following medical terms related to healthcare professions. You might need to refer to a medical dictionary for research.*

1. asthma: _____

2. eczema: _____

3. sinusitis: _____

4. prognosis: _____

5. biomonitoring: _____

Healthcare Professional Identification

Instructions: *Identify which of the appropriate healthcare professionals (allergist/immunologist, epidemiologist, oncology nurse) matches each of the following descriptions or tasks. You will use each profession more than once.*

1. may work at the CDC: _____

2. can order and interpret medical tests: _____

3. administers chemotherapy: _____

4. requires a degree from a medical school: _____

5. investigates how diseases are spread: _____

6. develops treatment plans for patients: _____

7. educates patients about home care: _____

8. performs statistical analysis on information about diseases: _____

9. works under the supervision of a physician: _____

Copyright Goodheart-Willcox Co., Inc.
May not be reproduced or posted to a publicly accessible website.

Chapter 7 Practice Test

Definitions

Instructions: *Use a regular or medical dictionary, or the Glossary/Index at the back of your textbook, to define the following terms.*

1. hemolysis: _____

2. splenomegaly: _____

3. antitoxin: _____

4. phlebitis: _____

5. thrombosis: _____

6. erythroblast: _____

7. fungal: _____

8. virologist: _____

9. metamorphosis: _____

10. phagocyte: _____

Build the Medical Term

Instructions: *Use the combining forms and suffixes listed on pages 173–175 of your textbook to build the medical term that corresponds to each of the following definitions.*

1. Word part: -ation
   Definition: process of clumping together

   Term: _____

2. Word part: -cyte
   Definition: cell with a large nucleus

   Term: _____

3. Word part: -plasm
   Definition: new formation/structure

   Term: _____

4. Word part: hem/a
   Definition: specialist in the study of blood

   Term: _____

5. Word part: -ical
   Definition: pertaining to the study of disease

   Term: _____

Copyright Goodheart-Willcox Co., Inc.
May not be reproduced or posted to a publicly accessible website.

Medical Terms and Definitions

Instructions: *Break down each of the following medical terms into its words parts (prefix, root word, combining vowel, and suffix if used). Then define each term.*

1. polymorphonuclear leukocyte

    Breakdown: _____

    Define: _____

2. fungology

    Breakdown: _____

    Define: _____

3. erythrocytopenia

    Breakdown: _____

    Define: _____

4. antineoplastic

    Breakdown: _____

    Define: _____

Review

Instructions: *Answer the following questions.*

1. List the three main types of cells in the blood.

    _____

    _____

    _____

2. Which term describes the type of immunity with which you were born?

    _____

3. Which term describes the condition in which a clotting protein is missing from the blood?

    _____

4. Why is mononucleosis called the *kissing disease*?

    _____

    _____

    _____

Copyright Goodheart-Willcox Co., Inc.
May not be reproduced or posted to a publicly accessible website.

CHAPTER 8 The Respiratory System

Activity A   Understanding Word Parts

Word Parts Matching, Part 1

Instructions: *Match each of the following word parts with the correct meaning.*

1. _____ voice
2. _____ dilation; expansion
3. _____ in; within
4. _____ painful; difficult
5. _____ pertaining to
6. _____ breathing
7. _____ carbon dioxide
8. _____ good; normal
9. _____ surgical opening
10. _____ chest; pleural cavity

A. dys-
B. eu-
C. -capnia
D. -thorax
E. -pnea
F. endo-
G. -tic
H. -phonia
I. -stomy
J. -ectasis

Word Parts Matching, Part 2

Instructions: *Match each of the following word parts with the correct meaning.*

1. _____ nose
2. _____ bronchial tube; bronchus
3. _____ pleura; serous membrane that enfolds the lungs
4. _____ air sac; alveolus
5. _____ sinus; cavity
6. _____ breathing
7. _____ to enlarge; expand
8. _____ oxygen
9. _____ cancer
10. _____ pus

A. dilat/o
B. py/o
C. spir/o
D. ox/i
E. alveol/o
F. bronch/o
G. sinus/o
H. pleur/o
I. rhin/o
J. carcin/o

Copyright Goodheart-Willcox Co., Inc.
May not be reproduced or posted to a publicly accessible website.

Build the Medical Term

Instructions: *Use the combining forms and suffixes listed on pages 204–205 of your textbook to build the medical term that corresponds to each of the following definitions.*

1. Word part: bronch/o

   Definition: muscle contraction of a bronchial tube

   Term: _____

2. Word part: rhin/o

   Definition: condition of excessive discharge from the nose

   Term: _____

3. Word part: pneum/o

   Definition: condition of air in the chest, pleural space

   Term: _____

4. Word part: -ic

   Definition: pertaining to the diaphragm

   Term: _____

Medical Terms and Definitions

Instructions: *Break down each of the following medical terms into its word parts (prefix, root word, combining vowel, and suffix if used). Then define each term.*

1. dysphonia

   Breakdown: _____

   Define: _____

2. tracheostomy

   Breakdown: _____

   Define: _____

3. bronchiectasis

   Breakdown: _____

   Define: _____

4. pyothorax

   Breakdown: _____

   Define: _____

5. spirometer

   Breakdown: _____

   Define: _____

6. thoracotomy

   Breakdown: _____

   Define: _____

Copyright Goodheart-Willcox Co., Inc.
May not be reproduced or posted to a publicly accessible website.

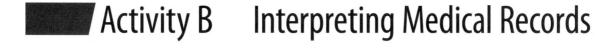

Activity B   Interpreting Medical Records

Medical Record Interpretation

Instructions: *Read the following medical record. Identify the meaning of the abbreviations and medical terms that appear in bold and are listed after the record. Refer to the table on page 228, Appendix B, and the Glossary/Index in the back of your textbook. Then answer the questions that follow.*

Medical Record

West Side ENT Clinic

Dictated by E. West, MD

Estella is a 3 **y/o** female with a history of chronic ear infections, allergic **rhinitis**, and **hypertrophy** of the tonsils and adenoids. She was referred to an **otorhinolaryngologist** for evaluation and **tx** recommendations. Pt's last tx for **tonsillitis** was 3 weeks ago. Strep test was negative. She was treated with Augmentin x 14 days.

Objective Data

General: Well-developed, well-nourished toddler. Responded adequately to age-appropriate commands.

GI: Pt's mother reports that Pt has a healthy appetite and normal bowel movements.

GU: Deferred

CV: heart sounds and rate **WNL** for age

Respiratory: Lungs clear to **auscultation**. No coughing or wheezing noted.

HEENT: PERRLA, denies **HA**, no gross abnormalities noted on external exam. No **lymphadenopathy** noted on **palpation** of posterior and anterior **cervical** lines. Pt is a mouth breather secondary to severe rhinitis. Tonsils are reddened, 3+ in size, and are crowding the **oropharyngeal** airway. Pt's mother confirms occasional **sleep apnea**, especially when Pt's allergy symptoms are severe. External ear canals are clean. Moderate bulging of the **tympanic membrane** is noted.

Recommendation: Schedule Pt for **tonsillectomy**, **adenoidectomy**, and **bilateral myringotomy** with placement of pressure-equalizing tubes.

1. y/o: _____

2. rhinitis: _____

3. hypertrophy: _____

4. otorhinolaryngologist: _____

5. tx: _____

6. tonsillitis: _____

7. GI: _____

8. CV: _____

9. WNL: _____

10. auscultation: _____

11. HEENT: _____

12. PERRLA: _____

13. HA: _____

14. lymphadenopathy: _____

15. palpation: _____

16. cervical: _____

17. oropharyngeal: _____

18. sleep apnea:_____

19. tympanic membrane: _____

20. tonsillectomy: _____

21. adenoidectomy:_____

22. myringotomy: _____

Review

Instructions: *Answer the following questions related to Estella's medical record.*

1. Where did the doctor check for swollen lymph nodes?

   _____

   _____

2. Why do you think this patient had occasional sleep apnea?

   _____

   _____

   _____

   _____

3. Refer to Figure 8.4 and the description of the pharynx and larynx on page 209 of your textbook. Why do you think a nasal infection can lead to an ear infection?

   _____

   _____

   _____

   _____

Copyright Goodheart-Willcox Co., Inc.
May not be reproduced or posted to a publicly accessible website.

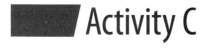 **Activity C** **Comprehending Anatomy and Physiology Terminology**

Review, Part 1

Instructions: *Answer the following questions.*

1. List the three main functions of the respiratory system.

   _____

2. Why do healthcare professionals usually measure a patient's respiratory rate after they measure the patient's pulse rate?

   _____

   _____

3. When a person suffers from an upper respiratory tract infection, which organs and structures may be affected?

   _____

4. Which structures in the vestibular region of the nasal cavities act as a first line of defense against infection?

   _____

Defining Terms

Instructions: *Define the following anatomical terms, and then use these terms to label the diagram that follows.*

1. nasopharynx:_____

2. oropharynx:_____

3. laryngopharynx: _____

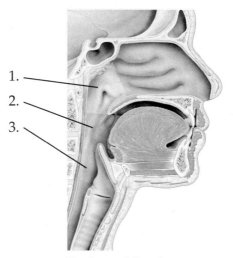

Regions of the pharynx

© *Body Scientific International*

1. Item 1:_____

2. Item 2:_____

3. Item 3:_____

Copyright Goodheart-Willcox Co., Inc.
May not be reproduced or posted to a publicly accessible website.

Review, Part 2

Instructions: *Answer the following questions.*

1. What is the purpose of the epiglottis?

   _____

   _____

   _____

2. What structures are considered to be part of the lower respiratory tract?

   _____

   _____

3. What does the term *ciliated* mean?

   _____

   _____

4. What does the term *bifurcate* mean?

   _____

   _____

5. In which respiratory structures does gas exchange occur?

   _____

6. Which term describes the structure that separates the thoracic cavity from the abdominal cavity?

   _____

7. Which term describes the watery membrane that surrounds the lungs?

   _____

8. Which term describes the fluid found between the two membranes of the lungs that reduces friction during inhalation and exhalation to make breathing easier?

   _____

9. Where is the control center that causes the diaphragm to contract, allowing air to flow into the lungs?

   _____

10. The level of what substance in the blood determines the rate of respirations?

    _____

Copyright Goodheart-Willcox Co., Inc.
May not be reproduced or posted to a publicly accessible website.

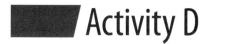 **Activity D   Understanding Terms Related to Diseases and Conditions**

Terms Matching

Instructions: *Match each of the following medical terms with the correct meaning.*

1. _____ a breathing pattern that is too slow and shallow

2. _____ a breathing pattern that is slower than normal

3. _____ a temporary interruption of breathing

4. _____ a breathing pattern that is deeper than normal

5. _____ a breathing pattern that is labored, difficult, or painful

6. _____ the term used to describe crackling sounds heard in the lungs

7. _____ a breathing pattern that is faster and deeper than normal

8. _____ a breathing pattern that is faster than normal

9. _____ the term used to describe coarse rattling or high-pitched snoring sounds heard in the lungs

10. _____ the term used to describe the harsh, high-pitched sound heard during inspiration

A. dyspnea

B. rales

C. hyperventilation

D. apnea

E. stridor

F. hyperpnea

G. tachypnea

H. bradypnea

I. rhonchi

J. hypoventilation

Scenarios

Instructions: *Read the following scenarios and answer the questions that follow.*

Scenario: *Imagine you are the nurse responsible for admitting patients into the ER. The first patient you see during your shift is a 20 y/o male who arrives via ambulance after being injured during a fight. He was stabbed in the left lateral side of the thoracic cavity. Air is now leaking into the pleural cavity.*

1. What is the term for this condition?

   _____

2. When the trauma surgeon evaluates this patient, she discovers that the knife severed several veins in the area. Now blood is leaking into the patient's pleural cavity. Which term describes this condition?

   _____

Scenario: *The next patient is a 72 y/o male with a long history of smoking. He has been diagnosed with a chronic pulmonary disease in which the alveoli are larger than normal and have lost their elasticity.*

1. What diagnosis will you record on this patient's admission form?

   _____

2. This patient's PCP recently told him that his lung function has worsened. His lungs' ability to perform their function of ventilation has been reduced, and he now has less than 50 percent normal inspiratory capacity based on his last pulmonary function test. Given this information, what additional diagnosis will you include on this patient's admission form?

   _____

Copyright Goodheart-Willcox Co., Inc.
May not be reproduced or posted to a publicly accessible website.

Scenario: *The next patient is Amy, a 7 y/o female who comes into the ER with c/o increased dyspnea. Her mother reports that Amy was playing outside earlier today while her neighbor was mowing the lawn. When Amy came into the house, her eyes were reddened and she had severe rhinorrhea. Amy told her mother that she could not breathe through her nose. Her mother says that the mucous membranes in Amy's nose were swollen and red.*

1. What diagnosis would you record in Amy's chart?

   _____

2. When you perform auscultation of Amy's lungs, you notice a definite wheezing sound during respiration. You know that this sound is made when there is a swelling or spasm of the bronchial tubes. What additional diagnosis do you now suspect for Amy?

   _____

Scenario: *Your next patient is Bobby, a 12 y/o male who c/o a sore throat. Upon examination of this patient, you notice that his tonsils are extremely inflamed.*

1. What is the medical term for this condition?

   _____

2. The ER doctor performs a test that confirms the presence of the bacterium *Streptococcus*. What diagnosis do you think matches Bobby's condition?

   _____

Copyright Goodheart-Willcox Co., Inc.
May not be reproduced or posted to a publicly accessible website.

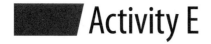 **Activity E   Analyzing Diagnostic-
and Treatment-Related Terms**

Instructions: *Answer the question in each of the following scenarios.*

1. One of your family members has been complaining that their significant other snores so loudly it keeps them up at night. Their significant other agrees to see the doctor because they have not been sleeping well either. The doctor orders a test to determine if your family member's significant other has sleep apnea. What is the name of this test?

   _____

2. If your family member's significant other is diagnosed with sleep apnea, they may receive treatment that includes wearing a mask attached to a machine that delivers mild air pressure to keep their airways open while they sleep. What is the name for this treatment method?

   _____

3. Your friend is a nurse's aide in a long-term skilled nursing facility. She tells you about a test that she had to have completed before she could work there. This test required her to have a small amount of a certain purified protein derivative injected under the skin of her forearm. She had to go back to the doctor's office 48–72 hours after the injection to see if there was any reaction to the derivative. What is the name of this test?

   _____

4. Your best friend's dad went to the doctor recently because he had a cough for about two weeks. The doctor suspects a diagnosis of pneumonia. What radiographic test might the doctor order to obtain images of the anterior, posterior, and lateral views of the lungs?

   _____

5. If the test mentioned in the previous question confirms that your friend's dad has pneumonia, the doctor may order another test. This test would determine which bacteria is growing in the lung secretions, as well as which antibiotic would most effectively treat the infection. What is the name of this test?

   _____

6. This test confirms that your friend's dad has bacterial pneumonia. What medication might the doctor prescribe to treat this infection?

   _____

7. You notice that you haven't seen your neighbor, Mr. Smith, out in his yard for several weeks. He used to stand on the front porch every night to smoke. When you next see Mrs. Smith, you ask about her husband, and she tells you that he is in the hospital. Mr. Smith started coughing up blood, so his wife took him to the hospital, where his PCP referred him to a cancer specialist. The pulmonary oncologist thinks that Mr. Smith may have bronchogenic carcinoma. Which test would the doctor order to examine lung secretions under a microscope to determine the presence of malignant cells?

   _____

8. Mr. Smith is confirmed to have cancer. The thoracic surgeon determines that there is a buildup of fluid in the pleural sac surrounding the affected lung. The surgeon schedules Mr. Smith for a procedure in which the fluid will be aspirated from this area. What is the term for this procedure?

   _____

Copyright Goodheart-Willcox Co., Inc.
May not be reproduced or posted to a publicly accessible website.

9. A week after this procedure is performed, the surgeon notices that fluid is continuing to build up in the area. This time, the surgeon recommends the placement of a chest tube that will drain the area. What is this procedure called?

_____

10. The surgeon orders a test to measure the amount of oxygen and carbon dioxide in Mr. Smith's blood. What is the name of this test?

_____

11. This test confirms that Mr. Smith's oxygen level is too low. What might the doctor order to help increase Mr. Smith's blood oxygen levels?

_____

12. You are enjoying a burger with your friends. You notice the man at the table next to you is eating and laughing loudly. Suddenly the man stops talking, puts his hands up to his throat, and tries to talk. You realize that this man's airway is obstructed and he is choking. What procedure must be performed on this man to clear his airway?

_____

13. You are outside mowing the lawn. You see your neighbor, Mr. Green, getting ready to run. Suddenly he falls to the ground. When you go to check on him, he is unresponsive. You notice that he is not breathing and does not have a heartbeat. You have been trained in an emergency lifesaving treatment that will attempt to restore normal cardiac and pulmonary functions. What is the name of this treatment?

_____

14. The emergency medical technicians arrive and take Mr. Green to the hospital in an ambulance. When you go to visit him later that day, you find out that the ER doctor put him on a machine that delivers artificial respirations because he is unable to breathe on his own. What is the name of this machine?

_____

15. To put Mr. Green on this machine, the ER doctor had to insert a breathing tube through his mouth and glottis, into the trachea. What is the name of this procedure?

_____

Copyright Goodheart-Willcox Co., Inc.
May not be reproduced or posted to a publicly accessible website.

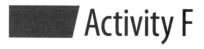 ## Activity F   Preparing for Your Future in Healthcare

Word Parts Matching

Instructions: *Match each of the following word parts with the correct meaning.*

1. _____ breathing

2. _____ surgical puncture to remove fluid

3. _____ to revive

4. _____ process of cutting; incision

5. _____ heart

6. _____ measure

7. _____ surgical opening

8. _____ lung

9. _____ process of measuring

A. cardi/o

B. pulmon/o

C. resuscit/o

D. spir/o

E. -centesis

F. -meter

G. -metry

H. –stomy

I. -tomy

Definitions

Instructions: *Refer to the description of healthcare professionals on page 229 of your textbook. Then define the following terms. You may use the information in your textbook, a regular or medical dictionary, the Glossary/Index in the back of your textbook, and your own words to define the terms.*

1. asthma: _____

_____

_____

_____

2. cerebrovascular accident: _____

_____

_____

_____

3. ventilator: _____

_____

_____

_____

4. thoracic cage: _____

_____

_____

_____

Copyright Goodheart-Willcox Co., Inc.
May not be reproduced or posted to a publicly accessible website.

5. lobectomy: _____

_____

_____

_____

6. pulmonary function test: _____

_____

_____

_____

7. endotracheal intubation: _____

_____

_____

_____

Healthcare Professional Identification

Instructions: *Identify the appropriate healthcare professional (respiratory therapist, perfusionist, pulmonologist, thoracic surgeon) that matches each of the following descriptions or tasks. You will use each profession more than once.*

1. requires a medical degree: _____

2. may care for patients in their homes: _____

3. performs surgery: _____

4. part of the surgical team in the operating room for heart and lung surgeries: _____

5. manages patients on ventilators: _____

6. cares for patients in intensive care centers: _____

7. manages the heart-lung machine: _____

8. may work in a nursing home or long-term care facility: _____

9. can administer blood products and medications: _____

Copyright Goodheart-Willcox Co., Inc.
May not be reproduced or posted to a publicly accessible website.

◢ Chapter 8 Practice Test

Definitions

Instructions: *Using the word parts on pages 204–205 and in Appendix A of your textbook, define the following medical terms.*

1. rhinoplasty: _____

2. bronchoscopy: _____

3. laryngectomy: _____

4. hemoptysis: _____

Medical Terms and Definitions

Instructions: *Break down each of the following medical terms into its word parts (prefix, root word, combining vowel, and suffix if used). Then define each term.*

1. pneumonia

   Breakdown: _____

   Define: _____

2. pneumonomelanosis

   Breakdown: _____

   Define: _____

3. pneumonomycosis

   Breakdown: _____

   Define: _____

4. laryngalgia

   Breakdown: _____

   Define: _____

5. endotracheal

   Breakdown: _____

   Define: _____

6. bronchorrhaphy

   Breakdown: _____

   Define: _____

7. pleurodynia

   Breakdown: _____

   Define: _____

Copyright Goodheart-Willcox Co., Inc.
May not be reproduced or posted to a publicly accessible website.

Review

Instructions: *Answer the following questions.*

1. Which gas is contained in the air that we breathe out?

    _____

2. When taking a patient's vital signs, what is considered one respiration?

    _____

3. What is considered a normal respiratory rate for a 16 y/o male?

    _____

4. What substance makes up the larynx and enables the vocal cords to move and produce sound?

    _____

Matching: Breathing

Instructions: *Match each of the following breathing-related medical terms with the correct meaning.*

1. _____ normal breathing

2. _____ fast breathing

3. _____ without breathing

4. _____ deep breathing

5. _____ difficult breathing

6. _____ straight breathing

7. _____ slow breathing

A. apnea

B. bradypnea

C. dyspnea

D. eupnea

E. hyperpnea

F. orthopnea

G. tachypnea

Matching: Diseases and Conditions

Instructions: *Match each of the following diseases and conditions with the correct meaning.*

1. _____ a traveling blood clot that becomes lodged in a lung

2. _____ childhood disease characterized by a "barking" cough

3. _____ condition of a collapsed or airless lung

4. _____ congenital disease that causes increased production of mucus in the lungs

5. _____ the result of excessive fluid buildup in the pleural cavity

6. _____ inflammation of the throat

7. _____ the presence of pus in the pleural cavity

8. _____ the presence of blood in the pleural cavity

A. pleural effusion

B. empyema

C. hemothorax

D. croup

E. pulmonary embolism

F. cystic fibrosis

G. atelectasis

H. pharyngitis

Copyright Goodheart-Willcox Co., Inc.
May not be reproduced or posted to a publicly accessible website.

CHAPTER 9 | The Digestive System

Activity A   Understanding Word Parts

Word Parts Matching, Part 1

Instructions: *Match each of the following word parts with the correct meaning.*

1. _____ abdominal wall; abdomen
2. _____ gallbladder
3. _____ rectum; anus
4. _____ stomach
5. _____ sugar
6. _____ bile; gall
7. _____ intestines
8. _____ tooth
9. _____ colon; large intestine
10. _____ groin

A. enter/o
B. col/o
C. bil/i
D. gastr/o
E. inguin/o
F. gluc/o
G. lapar/o
H. proct/o
I. dent/i
J. cholecyst/o

Word Parts Matching, Part 2

Instructions: *Match each of the following word parts with the correct meaning.*

1. _____ vomiting
2. _____ complete; through
3. _____ surgical opening
4. _____ before; in front of
5. _____ meal
6. _____ defecation; elimination of waste
7. _____ flow; excessive discharge
8. _____ appetite
9. _____ around; surrounding
10. _____ digestion

A. peri-
B. -chezia
C. pre-
D. -pepsia
E. dia-
F. -rrhea
G. -stomy
H. -orexia
I. -prandial
J. -emesis

Copyright Goodheart-Willcox Co., Inc.
May not be reproduced or posted to a publicly accessible website.

Build the Medical Term

Instructions: *Use the combining forms, prefixes, and suffixes listed on pages 235–236 of your textbook to build the medical term that corresponds to each of the following definitions.*

1. Word part: col/o

   Definition: creation of a surgical opening in the colon

   Term: _____

2. Word part: lapar/o

   Definition: instrument used to view the abdomen

   Term: _____

3. Word part: an-

   Definition: condition of without an appetite

   Term: _____

4. Word part: -prandial

   Definition: after a meal

   Term: _____

Medical Terms and Definitions

Instructions: *Break down each of the following medical terms into its word parts (prefix, root word, combining vowel, and suffix if used). Then define each term.*

1. gastroenteritis

   Breakdown: _____

   Define: _____

2. cholecystectomy

   Breakdown: _____

   Define: _____

3. oropharyngeal

   Breakdown: _____

   Define: _____

4. periodontist

   Breakdown: _____

   Define: _____

5. lithotripsy

   Breakdown: _____

   Define: _____

6. gingivectomy

   Breakdown: _____

   Define: _____

Copyright Goodheart-Willcox Co., Inc.
May not be reproduced or posted to a publicly accessible website.

Name _____

Activity B   Interpreting Medical Records

Instructions: *Read the medical records that follow. Identify the meaning of the abbreviations that appear in bold and are listed after each record, and then answer the question that follows.*

Medical Record A

Notes from Dr. Orr, **ATT PHYS**, **GI** specialist to **RN**
Schedule **Pt** for an **OP EGD** and **colonoscopy**. Pt has **hx** of **GERD**. Remind Pt to be **n.p.o.** 12 hours prior to procedure.

1. ATT PHYS: _____

2. GI: _____

3. RN: _____

4. Pt: _____

5. OP: _____

6. EGD: _____

7. colonoscopy: _____

8. hx: _____

9. GERD: _____

10. n.p.o.: _____

11. Why do you think this patient is ordered to be n.p.o. prior to the procedure?

_____

_____

Medical Record B

Notes from B. Kramer, Doctor of **Dental** Surgery to dental assistant
Set up appointment for Pt to see Dr. S. Adams, a specialist in **oral** surgery, to evaluate for possible **hemiglossectomy** because of oral cancer. Remind Pt to take his recent **CAT** scan films to the appointment. Instruct Pt that he will be discharged to home with a **NG** tube for nutritional support.

1. Dental: _____

2. oral: _____

3. hemiglossectomy: _____

4. CAT: _____

5. NG: _____

6. Why do you think this patient will need the NG tube after surgery?

_____

_____

Copyright Goodheart-Willcox Co., Inc.
May not be reproduced or posted to a publicly accessible website.

Medical Record C

Notes from T. Ayers, **ER** Physician Assistant, to pt's **PCP**, Dr. R. Bailey
Pt was evaluated in ER with **c/o** chest tightness, **SOB**, and **dyspepsia**. Pt was concerned that he was having an **MI**. **P** and **BP** were **WNL**. **Lab** test for **cardiac** enzymes and **EKG** to **R/O** MI was negative. **UGI** X-rays **Dx** a hiatal hernia. Instructed Pt to take **OTC** antacids **p.r.n.** 1 hour **p.c.** and at **hs**. Please follow up with pt for further **tx**.

1. ER: _____

2. PCP: _____

3. c/o: _____

4. SOB: _____

5. dyspepsia: _____

6. MI: _____

7. P: _____

8. BP: _____

9. WNL: _____

10. lab: _____

11. cardiac: _____

12. EKG: _____

13. R/O: _____

14. UGI: _____

15. Dx: _____

16. OTC: _____

17. p.r.n.: _____

18. p.c.: _____

19. hs: _____

20. tx: _____

21. Why might this patient have thought he was having an MI when he went into the ER?

_____

_____

_____

_____

Copyright Goodheart-Willcox Co., Inc.
May not be reproduced or posted to a publicly accessible website.

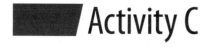 Activity C   Comprehending Anatomy
and Physiology Terminology

Definitions

Instructions: *Use a regular or medical dictionary, the Glossary/Index in the back of your textbook, and your own words to define the following terms.*

1. ingestion

_____

_____

2. absorption

_____

_____

3. buccae

_____

_____

4. gingiva

_____

_____

5. deglutition

_____

_____

Review

Instructions: *Answer the following questions.*

1. What is the function of bile?

_____

_____

_____

2. What makes it possible for some medications to be absorbed under the tongue?

_____

_____

_____

3. What is the function of the enzyme you named in the previous question?

_____

_____

_____

Copyright Goodheart-Willcox Co., Inc.
May not be reproduced or posted to a publicly accessible website.

4. Which term describes the ring-like muscle at the end of the esophagus that controls the flow of substances?

_____

5. Which term describes the upper part of the stomach?

_____

Terms Matching

Instructions: *Match each of the following terms, which are related to a part of the intestine, with the correct meaning.*

1. _____ pouch that connects to the distal end of the ileum

2. _____ section of the large intestine that starts at the cecum and ends below the liver

3. _____ twelve-foot section of the small intestine where vitamin B_{12} is absorbed

4. _____ part of the large intestine that is named because of its shape

5. _____ first section of the small intestine, where absorption of nutrients begins

6. _____ section of the large intestine that starts on the left lateral side of the body and ends in the left inferior portion of the abdominal cavity

7. _____ the middle section of the small intestine, which measures about 8 feet in length

8. _____ storage area for feces

9. _____ appendage of the cecum that has no known function

10. _____ the longest section of the large intestine

A. duodenum

B. jejunum

C. ileum

D. cecum

E. appendix

F. ascending colon

G. transverse colon

H. descending colon

I. sigmoid colon

J. rectum

Large Intestine Identification

Instructions: *Label the different sections of the large intestine in the following image.*

1. Item 1:_____

2. Item 2:_____

3. Item 3:_____

4. Item 4:_____

5. Item 5:_____

6. Item 6:_____

7. Item 7:_____

8. Item 8:_____

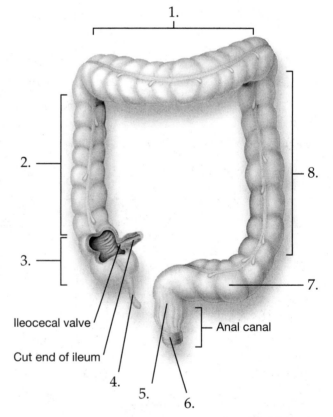

Ileocecal valve

Cut end of ileum

Anal canal

© *Body Scientific International*

Copyright Goodheart-Willcox Co., Inc.
May not be reproduced or posted to a publicly accessible website.

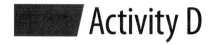 **Activity D   Understanding Terms Related to Diseases and Conditions**

Define Word Parts

Instructions: *Using the information on pages 235–236 of your textbook, define the following word parts.*

1. -orexia: _____

2. appendic/o: _____

3. chol/e: _____

4. cirrh/o: _____

5. dent/i: _____

6. hepat/o: _____

7. inguin/o: _____

8. pancreat/o: _____

9. odont/o: _____

Matching

Instructions: *Match each of the following medical terms with the correct meaning.*

1. _____ condition in which the upper part of the stomach protrudes through the esophageal opening in the diaphragm

2. _____ condition involving self-deprivation of food and pathological weight loss

3. _____ inflammation of the abdominal cavity

4. _____ tooth decay that leads to cavities

5. _____ inflammation of the appendix

6. _____ inflammation of the liver, generally caused by a viral infection

7. _____ scarring of the liver, generally caused by alcohol and/or drug abuse or chronic liver inflammation

8. _____ chronic inflammation of the colon with ulcers

9. _____ abnormal twisting of the intestines

10. _____ swollen, twisted veins in the lower end of the esophagus

A. volvulus
B. anorexia nervosa
C. peritonitis
D. dental caries
E. esophageal varices
F. hiatal hernia
G. ulcerative colitis
H. hepatitis
I. cirrhosis
J. appendicitis

GI Disorder Terms

Instructions: *Choose the correct term for each sign or symptom of a GI disorder.*

1. _____ vomiting blood
A. hemoptysis
B. hematochezia
C. hematemesis
D. hemorrhage

Copyright Goodheart-Willcox Co., Inc.
May not be reproduced or posted to a publicly accessible website.

2. _____ painful or difficult swallowing
   A. dysphonia
   B. dysphagia
   C. dyspepsia
   D. dyspnea

3. _____ abnormal accumulation of fluid in the abdomen
   A. constipation
   B. cirrhosis
   C. diarrhea
   D. ascites

4. _____ yellow discoloration of the skin due to blood disorder
   A. cyanosis
   B. cirrhosis
   C. jaundice
   D. peritonitis

5. _____ bad breath
   A. flatus
   B. eructation
   C. jaundice
   D. halitosis

6. _____ unpleasant sensation in the stomach that causes an urge to vomit
   A. anorexia
   B. nausea
   C. emesis
   D. dyspepsia

7. _____ the backward flow of food into the esophagus
   A. regurgitation
   B. dyspepsia
   C. dysphagia
   D. borborygmus

8. _____ lack of appetite
   A. nausea
   B. emesis
   C. regurgitation
   D. anorexia

9. _____ movement of gas in the digestive tract that makes rumbling sounds in the abdomen
   A. borborygmus
   B. flatus
   C. regurgitation
   D. emesis

Copyright Goodheart-Willcox Co., Inc.
May not be reproduced or posted to a publicly accessible website.

Name _____

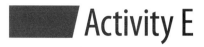 **Activity E   Analyzing Diagnostic-
                      and Treatment-Related Terms**

Instructions: *Read the following scenarios and answer the question for each one.*

1. Mr. Barker is a 51 y/o male. His father died at age 68 of colon cancer. Mr. Barker's PCP performed an office procedure in which only the sigmoid colon was examined using a scope. What is the name of this test?

_____

2. Mr. Barker's PCP referred him to a GI specialist, Dr. Miller, to be evaluated for colon cancer. Dr. Miller recommended that Mr. Barker undergo a test to visually examine the colon with a scope. What is the name of this test?

_____

3. During the procedure, Dr. Miller noticed a colon polyp in the distal end of the descending colon. The doctor removed the entire polyp and gave it to the nurse to be evaluated under a microscope to see if it is cancerous. What is the name of this test?

_____

4. Dr. Miller decided to order further testing on Mr. Barker. He ordered a test in which barium (a contrast agent) is put into the rectum and X-rays are taken of the lower part of the digestive tract. What is the name of this test?

_____

5. Mr. Rodriguez is a 62 y/o male who noticed some bright red blood in the toilet after going to the bathroom. He contacted his PCP, Dr. Pena. Which term might Mr. Rodriguez use to describe this symptom?

_____

6. Before Mr. Rodriguez came into the office, Dr. Pena wanted him to take a sample of his feces to the laboratory. At the laboratory, healthcare professionals evaluated the sample to see if there was any blood present. What is the name of this test?

_____

7. Dr. Pena had Mr. Rodriguez come into the office so he could perform a visual examination of the rectum using a scope. What is the name of this test?

_____

8. Mrs. Thomas visited the radiology department of the hospital, where she was scheduled to have a test that uses sound waves to generate an image of the abdominal organs. During this test, healthcare professionals will check her gallbladder to see if stones are present. What is the name of this test?

_____

9. If there are stones in Mrs. Thomas' gallbladder, what term would a healthcare professional use to describe her condition?

_____

10. Miss Davis has been experiencing stomach pain for several months. Her doctor ordered a blood test to see if she has the bacteria known as *H. pylori* in her body. What is the name of this test?

_____

11. Mr. Stevens has been having problems swallowing. His doctor ordered a test in which Mr. Stevens drinks a substance that will show up on a specialized X-ray. Pictures are taken while Mr. Stevens is swallowing the substance so that the doctor can evaluate his swallowing mechanism. What is the name of this test?

_____

Copyright Goodheart-Willcox Co., Inc.
May not be reproduced or posted to a publicly accessible website.

12. Which medical term describes the problem that Mr. Stevens is experiencing?

_____

13. Clare is a nurse practitioner in an outpatient drug and alcohol treatment center. One of the patients she cares for has been complaining of right upper abdominal pain. Clare is concerned that this patient may have a condition that involves scarring of the liver. She ordered a blood test that will measure the different enzymes used in the function of the liver. What is the name of this test?

_____

14. Which term describes the medical condition that Clare suspects this patient has?

_____

15. Deidre is a 45 y/o female with complaints of epigastric pain. A physician assistant in the clinic referred her to a GI specialist to have several tests performed. One of the tests will take place in the radiology department of the hospital. Deidre will be given barium to drink, and then X-rays of her stomach and duodenum will be taken. What is the name of this test?

_____

16. Deidre is also scheduled to have a test performed in which the GI specialist will put a fiber-optic scope in her mouth, down the esophagus, to the stomach, and into the duodenum. What is the name of this test?

_____

17. Describe where Deidre's *epigastric* pain is located.

_____

18. Chloe is a 16 y/o female who has been receiving chemotherapy treatment for leukemia. She has been experiencing some side effects of the treatment, including anorexia and hyperemesis. Describe what the term *hyperemesis* means.

_____

19. What type of medication might the doctor give Chloe to help relieve her hyperemesis?

_____

20. Heather is a 26 y/o who has had problems with weight management since she was in high school. She has tried dieting and exercise but has been unable to lose weight. She is considering having surgery that will reduce the size of her stomach. What is this type of surgery called?

_____

Copyright Goodheart-Willcox Co., Inc.
May not be reproduced or posted to a publicly accessible website.

◢ Activity F   Preparing for Your Future in Healthcare

Instructions: *Identify the appropriate healthcare professional (dental hygienist, dentist, gastroenterologist, registered dietitian) that matches each of the following scenarios. You will use each profession more than once.*

1. A professional model who noticed a stain on her front tooth contacts this healthcare professional to have the stain removed.

   _____

2. A 42 y/o male with pain and swelling in his left lower jaw for three days saw his primary care physician, who said he has an abscessed (infected) tooth that may need to be pulled. The PCP refers her patient to this healthcare professional.

   _____

3. A 25 y/o pregnant female has been diagnosed with gestational diabetes. Her OB/GYN wants her to meet with this healthcare professional to help develop a diet plan to follow during her pregnancy.

   _____

4. A 23 y/o female college student has been experiencing diarrhea for several days, followed by constipation. She also reports bloating, abdominal cramping, and weight loss. The nurse practitioner (NP) who has been seeing this patient is concerned that she has irritable bowel syndrome. The NP will refer her to this specialist for treatment options.

   _____

5. A 12 y/o male has a fractured tooth after being hit in the face with a softball. His mom calls this healthcare professional to make an appointment for him.

   _____

6. A 54 y/o high school teacher needs to make his six-month follow-up appointment for a teeth cleaning. He would make an appointment with this healthcare professional.

   _____

7. A 45 y/o female comes into the local food pantry asking for help with meal planning. Her daughter was recently diagnosed with celiac disease, and she does not understand what kinds of foods her daughter should avoid. She is scared that her daughter will get sick again. The counselors at the food pantry would recommend the woman see this healthcare professional.

   _____

8. An 80 y/o female resident of a nursing home has not had a bowel movement in five days. When the resident says she needs to use the toilet, the nurse aide assists her. After the aide helps the resident back into her wheelchair, the aide notices bright red blood in the toilet. The aide reports this to his charge nurse. The charge nurse documents the occurrence of constipation and hematochezia in the resident's chart. The charge nurse would make an appointment with this healthcare professional for the resident.

   _____

Copyright Goodheart-Willcox Co., Inc.
May not be reproduced or posted to a publicly accessible website.

Chapter 9 Practice Test

Definitions

Instructions: *Using the word parts on pages 235–236 of your textbook, define the following medical terms.*

1. hyperemesis

_____

_____

2. hepatorrhaphy

_____

_____

3. cholecystalgia

_____

_____

4. dentalgia

_____

_____

5. nasogastric

_____

_____

Medical Terms and Definitions

Instructions: *Break down each of the following medical terms into its word parts (prefix, root word, combining vowel, and suffix if used). Then define each term.*

1. abdominocentesis

    Breakdown: _____

    Define: _____

2. colostomy

    Breakdown: _____

    Define: _____

3. hepatocyte

    Breakdown: _____

    Define: _____

4. pharyngoplasty

    Breakdown: _____

    Define: _____

Copyright Goodheart-Willcox Co., Inc.
May not be reproduced or posted to a publicly accessible website.

5. splenorrhaphy

   Breakdown: _____

   Define: _____

6. proctosigmoidoscopy

   Breakdown: _____

   Define: _____

Review

Instructions: *Answer the following questions.*

1. Which type of digestion involves saliva secreted by the salivary glands?

   _____

2. What is the purpose of the uvula?

   _____

3. Which term describes the mixture of partially digested food and gastric juices that passes from the stomach into the first section of the small intestine?

   _____

4. What is the largest internal organ in the body?

   _____

Disease or Condition Identification

Instructions: *Identify the term that corresponds to each disease or condition described below.*

1. a chronic disease that causes inflammation of the digestive tract and generally affects the ileum and the colon

   _____

2. a chronic viral infection that causes liver inflammation and damage and is usually transmitted by blood or body fluids during sexual contact or childbirth

   _____

3. a condition that occurs due to high levels of bilirubin in the blood

   _____

Copyright Goodheart-Willcox Co., Inc.
May not be reproduced or posted to a publicly accessible website.

Matching

Instructions: *Match each of the following terms with the correct meaning.*

1. _____ surgical opening of the large intestine

2. _____ drug used to stimulate defecation

3. _____ test that detects the presence of hidden blood in the feces

4. _____ laboratory test that detects the presence of pathogens in the blood

5. _____ laboratory test that measures the number and types of cells in the blood

6. _____ visual examination of the rectum using a scope

7. _____ visual examination of the digestive tract using a wireless camera

8. _____ X-ray of the large intestine and rectum using a contrast medium

9. _____ drug that prevents or relieves nausea and vomiting

10. _____ surgical procedure used to treat morbid obesity

A. proctoscopy
B. antiemetic
C. barium enema
D. capsule endoscopy
E. laxative
F. occult blood test
G. serology test
H. bariatric surgery
I. CBC
J. colostomy

Copyright Goodheart-Willcox Co., Inc.
May not be reproduced or posted to a publicly accessible website.

CHAPTER 10   The Nervous System and Mental Health

Activity A   Understanding Word Parts

Word Parts Matching, Part 1

Instructions: *Match each of the following word parts with the correct meaning.*

1. _____ hernia; swelling; protrusion
2. _____ speech
3. _____ to seize; take hold of
4. _____ below; under
5. _____ suture
6. _____ weakness
7. _____ pain; sensitivity
8. _____ hardening; thickening
9. _____ paralysis
10. _____ together; with

A. -paresis
B. -sclerosis
C. -rrhaphy
D. -phasia
E. -algesia
F. -cele
G. -plegia
H. -leptic
I. con-
J. sub-

Word Parts Matching, Part 2

Instructions: *Match each of the following word parts with the correct meaning.*

1. _____ speech
2. _____ brain
3. _____ glue
4. _____ head
5. _____ gray matter
6. _____ nerve root
7. _____ development; nourishment
8. _____ split
9. _____ coordination; order
10. _____ water

A. schiz/o
B. poli/o
C. hydr/o
D. radicul/o
E. troph/o
F. encephal/o
G. cephal/o
H. phas/o
I. tax/o
J. gli/o

Copyright Goodheart-Willcox Co., Inc.
May not be reproduced or posted to a publicly accessible website.

Build the Medical Term

Instructions: *Use the prefixes and suffixes listed on pages 273–275 of your textbook to build the medical term that corresponds to each of the following definitions.*

1. Word part: -al
   Definition: pertaining to fainting

   Term: _____

2. Word part: -algia
   Definition: nerve pain

   Term: _____

3. Word part: -ia
   Definition: condition of faulty or difficult speech

   Term: _____

4. Word part: -ia
   Definition: condition of difficulty with words

   Term: _____

5. Word part: -algia
   Definition: head pain (headache)

   Term: _____

6. Word part: an-
   Definition: without feeling or sensation

   Term: _____

Medical Terms and Definitions

Instructions: *Break down each of the following medical terms into its word parts (prefix, root word, combining vowel, and suffix if used). Then define each term.*

1. schizophrenia

   Breakdown: _____

   Define: _____

2. hydrocephalus

   Breakdown: _____

   Define: _____

3. meningocele

   Breakdown: _____

   Define: _____

4. ischemia

   Breakdown: _____

   Define: _____

Copyright Goodheart-Willcox Co., Inc.
May not be reproduced or posted to a publicly accessible website.

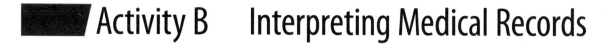 Activity B   Interpreting Medical Records

Instructions: *Read the medical records that follow. Identify the meaning of the abbreviations that appear in bold and are listed after the record, and then answer the following question.*

Medical Record A

20 y/o female college student with **PMH** of mild **CP** presents to on-campus medical clinic with **c/o** severe **HA**, fever, fatigue, and **photophobia**. Pt has a positive Babinski sign. Clinic physician assistant has ordered **LP** to collect and analyze sample of **CSF** to **R/O** bacterial **meningitis**.

1. PMH: _____

2. CP: _____

3. c/o: _____

4. HA: _____

5. photophobia: _____

_____

_____

6. LP: _____

7. CSF: _____

8. R/O: _____

9. meningitis: _____

_____

_____

10. What is the Babinski sign?

_____

_____

_____

_____

_____

_____

_____

Copyright Goodheart-Willcox Co., Inc.
May not be reproduced or posted to a publicly accessible website.

Medical Record B

72 y/o male admitted to **ER** by ambulance with c/o **dystaxia**, numbness on the **L** side of his face and arm, **dysphasia**, and **dysphagia**. Pt's wife states that he seemed to "black out" for about 30 seconds, and then fell onto the bed. She also stated that Pt saw his **PCP** last week and was **Dx** with **TIA**.

PE: left sided weakness noted

Plan: **MRI** head **STAT** to **R/O CVA**

1. ER: _____

2. dystaxia: _____

_____

_____

3. L: _____

4. dysphasia: _____

_____

_____

5. dysphagia: _____

_____

_____

6. PCP: _____

7. Dx: _____

8. TIA: _____

9. PE: _____

10. MRI: _____

11. STAT: _____

12. R/O: _____

13. CVA: _____

14. Why was the Dx of TIA important in this case?

_____

_____

_____

_____

_____

Copyright Goodheart-Willcox Co., Inc.
May not be reproduced or posted to a publicly accessible website.

Medical Record C

24 y/o male was transported to ER after being involved in a motorcycle accident. Pt was not wearing a helmet. **CT** shows **SDH**. MRI reveals **SCI**. Admitted to critical care unit to perform **EEG** and monitor **ICP**.

1. CT: _____

2. SDH: _____

3. SCI: _____

4. EEG: _____

5. ICP: _____

6. Explain where a SDH might be located.

_____

_____

_____

_____

Medical Record D

10 y/o male was referred by pediatrician to child psychiatry for evaluation due to poor grades and difficulty sitting in class. Pt's mother reports that pt has been getting into trouble at school. Pt's mother also reports that she and Pt's dad have recently divorced. Mental health specialist Dx Pt with **ADHD** and **GAD**. Recommends Pt undergo **OP CBT**.

1. ADHD: _____

2. GAD: _____

3. OP: _____

4. CBT: _____

5. What may be one cause of the Pt's GAD?

_____

_____

_____

_____

Copyright Goodheart-Willcox Co., Inc.
May not be reproduced or posted to a publicly accessible website.

Activity C   Comprehending Anatomy and Physiology Terminology

Definitions

Instructions: *Use a regular or medical dictionary, the Glossary/Index in the back of your textbook, and your own words to define the following terms.*

1. homeostasis:

   _____

   _____

2. neurons:

   _____

   _____

3. neuroglial cells:

   _____

   _____

4. sensory neurons:

   _____

   _____

5. motor neurons:

   _____

   _____

6. central nervous system:

   _____

   _____

7. peripheral nervous system:

   _____

   _____

8. reflex:

   _____

   _____

9. autonomic nervous system:

   _____

   _____

10. somatic nervous system:

   _____

   _____

Copyright Goodheart-Willcox Co., Inc.
May not be reproduced or posted to a publicly accessible website.

11. sympathetic nervous system:

_____

_____

12. parasympathetic nervous system:

_____

_____

Review

Instructions: *Answer the following questions.*

1. Which body system does the nervous system work closely with to help maintain homeostasis?

   _____

2. Which term describes changes in the internal or external environments that can cause a nervous system response?

   _____

3. What is the process by which the central nervous system interprets all the information it receives from organs such as the eyes and the skin?

   _____

4. Which division of the nervous system makes voluntary movement possible?

   _____

5. Which term describes the process of transmitting nerve impulses from the brain and spinal cord to all other parts of the body?

   _____

6. What is the difference between gray matter and white matter?

   _____

7. Which term describes the connective tissues that surround the CNS?

   _____

Terms Matching

Instructions: *Match each of the following terms related to the brain with the correct meaning.*

1. _____ area of the brain that processes stimuli related to touch and pain

2. _____ convolutions on the surface of the brain

3. _____ part of the brain that controls balance and equilibrium

4. _____ serves as the conduit for sensory information between the cerebrum or cerebellum and the rest of the body

5. _____ the largest region of the brain

6. _____ area of the brain that controls language processing

7. _____ area of the brain that controls hunger, thirst, and digestion

8. _____ area of the brain that is the "seat of your personality"

9. _____ the site of three key glands

10. _____ gland that secretes melatonin

A. cerebrum

B. gyri

C. frontal lobe

D. parietal lobe

E. temporal lobe

F. cerebellum

G. diencephalon

H. hypothalamus

I. pineal gland

J. brain stem

Copyright Goodheart-Willcox Co., Inc.
May not be reproduced or posted to a publicly accessible website.

Activity D   Understanding Terms Related to Diseases and Conditions

Matching

Instructions: *Match each of the following terms related to neurological conditions with the correct meaning.*

1. _____ paralysis of the lower half of the body

2. _____ involuntary trembling or shaking of the body or limbs

3. _____ disruption of the electrical activity of the brain

4. _____ a sensation that often occurs before a seizure or migraine

5. _____ sensation of numbness, prickling, or tingling

6. _____ diffuse pain in one or more parts of the head

7. _____ a state of extended unconsciousness

8. _____ a sudden, abnormal, involuntary contraction of the muscles

9. _____ fainting

10. _____ paralysis of one side of the body

A. aura
B. coma
C. convulsion
D. headache
E. hemiplegia
F. paraplegia
G. paresthesia
H. seizure
I. syncope
J. tremor

Medical Scenarios

Instructions: *Read the following scenarios and answer the question in each scenario.*

1. A 17-year-old linebacker for the high school football team had a helmet-to-helmet collision with the running back from the opposing team. The linebacker was assisted off the field and evaluated by the trainer, who recommended that he be evaluated in the emergency room. The MRI in the emergency room showed bruising of the cerebral tissue. What is the diagnosis for this patient?

_____

2. An abdominal ultrasound of a pregnant woman shows that her baby has a protrusion of the spinal cord and meninges. What is the baby's diagnosis?

_____

3. A 68-year-old man comes to the hospital because his wife has noticed he's having trouble holding things. He also walks slowly and has a difficult time walking in the store with his wife. When the doctor examines this man, she notices that his posture is more stooped than the last time he was examined, about six months earlier. What is the patient's diagnosis?

_____

4. A 43-year-old female was discharged from the hospital after spending almost two weeks there due to a severe respiratory viral infection. One week later, she returned to the emergency room with complaints of muscle pain and weakness that had gotten progressively worse since she was discharged from the hospital. She had also noticed that she lost voluntary movement of her fingers. What is this patient's diagnosis?

_____

Copyright Goodheart-Willcox Co., Inc.
May not be reproduced or posted to a publicly accessible website.

5. A 5-year-old male was admitted to the pediatric intensive care unit by his pediatrician because he developed symptoms of confusion and did not know who his mother was. He had two seizures on the way to the doctor's office and became unconscious. The pediatric neurologist also noticed that this patient has hepatomegaly. What is the patient's diagnosis?

_____

Mental Health Conditions

Instructions: *Choose the correct mental health condition for each of the following descriptions.*

1. _____ This developmental disability appears in childhood, and it is characterized by difficulty communicating and making eye contact with others, as well as repetitive motor activities, such as rocking back and forth.
   A. ADHD
   B. dyslexia
   C. ASD
   D. ID

2. _____ In this mental illness, a person will eat large amounts of food, and then purge through induced vomiting or use of laxatives. Excessive exercise may also occur.
   A. anorexia nervosa
   B. schizophrenia
   C. seasonal affective disorder
   D. bulimia nervosa

3. _____ This mood disorder is characterized by severe sadness and lack of interest in normal activities. Symptoms generally occur around the winter months.
   A. SAD
   B. bipolar disorder
   C. postpartum psychosis
   D. OCD

4. _____ In this anxiety disorder, a person will perform the same activity over and over, such as washing hands every hour even though the skin is dry, cracked, and extremely painful.
   A. panic disorder
   B. GAD
   C. PTSD
   D. OCD

5. _____ This mental illness is commonly seen in soldiers who return from war and in people who have experienced assault or abuse. People with this mental illness may experience exaggerated fears and difficulty sleeping.
   A. PD
   B. PTSD
   C. OCD
   D. GAD

6. _____ In this mental illness, people may be abnormally happy one day and so extremely sad the next day that they cannot get out of bed.
   A. SAD
   B. postpartum psychosis
   C. bipolar disorder
   D. schizophrenia

Copyright Goodheart-Willcox Co., Inc.
May not be reproduced or posted to a publicly accessible website.

Activity E   Analyzing Diagnostic- and Treatment-Related Terms

Definitions

Instructions: *Using the word parts on pages 273–275 of your textbook, define the following medical terms.*

1. ischemia: _____

_____

2. neuroleptic: _____

_____

3. hypnotic: _____

_____

4. anesthetic: _____

_____

5. subdural: _____

_____

6. anxiolytic: _____

_____

7. myelogram: _____

_____

8. craniectomy: _____

_____

Identifying Terms

Instructions: *Identify the term that corresponds to each diagnostic test or treatment method described.*

1. measures the speed at which electrical impulses travel through a nerve and can be used to diagnose carpal tunnel syndrome or myasthenia gravis:

_____

2. a record of the electrical impulses of the brain; useful in evaluating seizure disorders, strokes, and the brain function of patients in a coma:

_____

3. X-ray of the spinal cord that is useful in evaluating spinal tumors, herniated vertebral disks, or spinal stenosis:

_____

4. test in which the reflexes on the plantar surface of the foot are stimulated to assist in diagnosing neurological disorders such as brain tumors and meningitis:

_____

Copyright Goodheart-Willcox Co., Inc.
May not be reproduced or posted to a publicly accessible website.

5. two tests that can be performed to assist in diagnosing a CVA:

_____

6. test that involves collecting and evaluating CSF and can assist in diagnosing meningitis, Guillain-Barré syndrome, or cancers of the brain and spinal cord:

_____

7. pain-management procedure in which an anesthetic is injected into an area near a nerve:

_____

8. surgical repair of a nerve:

_____

9. surgical procedure in which the inner layer of a carotid artery is cleared of fatty plaque deposits to improve blood flow to the brain:

_____

10. surgical procedure that treats a herniated disk of the spine, in which all or part of the lamina of a vertebra is removed:

_____

11. procedure used to treat severe depression, in which electrical shocks are applied to the brain:

_____

Matching

Instructions: *Match each of the following types of drugs with the correct meaning.*

1. _____ causes a loss of sensation

2. _____ reduces feelings of anxiety

3. _____ promotes sleep and loss of consciousness

4. _____ relieves pain

5. _____ produces a soothing or tranquilizing effect

6. _____ treats convulsions

A. sedative

B. analgesic

C. anticonvulsant

D. hypnotic

E. anesthetic

F. anxiolytic

Copyright Goodheart-Willcox Co., Inc.
May not be reproduced or posted to a publicly accessible website.

Activity F   Preparing for Your Future in Healthcare

Define Word Parts

Instructions: *Use the information on pages 273–275 of your textbook to define the following word parts.*

1. crani/o: _____

2. dur/a: _____

3. encephal/o: _____

4. hypn/o: _____

5. neur/o: _____

6. psych/o: _____

7. traumat/o: _____

8. -esthesia: _____

9. -tomy: _____

10. -ectomy: _____

11. -ist: _____

12. -pathy: _____

Medical Terms and Definitions

Instructions: *Use a regular or medical dictionary, the glossary in the back of your textbook, and your own words to define the following terms.*

1. electroneurodiagnostic technician: _____

_____

_____

2. anesthetic: _____

_____

_____

3. hypnotic: _____

_____

_____

4. sedative: _____

_____

_____

Copyright Goodheart-Willcox Co., Inc.
May not be reproduced or posted to a publicly accessible website.

5. neuropathy: _____

_____

_____

6. epilepsy: _____

_____

_____

7. cerebrovascular accident: _____

_____

_____

8. aneurysm: _____

_____

_____

9. Parkinson's disease: _____

_____

_____

Identifying Healthcare Professionals

Instructions: *Identify the appropriate healthcare professional (anesthesiologist, electroneurodiagnostic technician, neurosurgeon) that matches each of the following descriptions or tasks. You will use each profession more than once, and some of the questions will have multiple answers.*

1. requires a medical degree: _____

2. may work in a sleep disorder lab: _____

3. may perform a craniotomy: _____

4. closely monitors a patient's heart rate: _____

5. requires a doctor's order to perform any test: _____

6. works in an operating room: _____

7. may repair an aneurysm: _____

8. administers drugs: _____

9. may perform an EEG: _____

Copyright Goodheart-Willcox Co., Inc.
May not be reproduced or posted to a publicly accessible website.

Chapter 10 Practice Test

Definitions

Instructions: *Using the word parts on pages 273–275 and Appendix A of your textbook, identify the medical term that corresponds to each of the following definitions.*

1. inflammation of the brain: _____

2. inflammation of the brain and spinal cord: _____

3. inflammation of the membranes around the brain and spinal cord: _____

4. paralysis of all four extremities: _____

5. disease of a nerve: _____

Medical Terms and Definitions

Instructions: *Break down each of the following medical terms into its word parts (prefix, root word, combining vowel, and suffix if used). Then define each term.*

1. encephalomyelopathy

   Breakdown: _____

   Define: _____

2. anesthesiologist

   Breakdown: _____

   Define: _____

3. radiculopathy

   Breakdown: _____

   Define: _____

4. hydrocephalus

   Breakdown: _____

   Define: _____

5. causalgia

   Breakdown: _____

   Define: _____

6. aphasia

   Breakdown: _____

   Define: _____

7. anencephaly

   Breakdown: _____

   Define: _____

Copyright Goodheart-Willcox Co., Inc.
May not be reproduced or posted to a publicly accessible website.

8. neuroma

　Breakdown: _____

　Define:_____

9. poliomyelitis

　Breakdown: _____

　Define:_____

10. cerebrovascular

　Breakdown: _____

　Define:_____

Brain Identification

Instructions: *Label the different parts of the brain in the following image.*

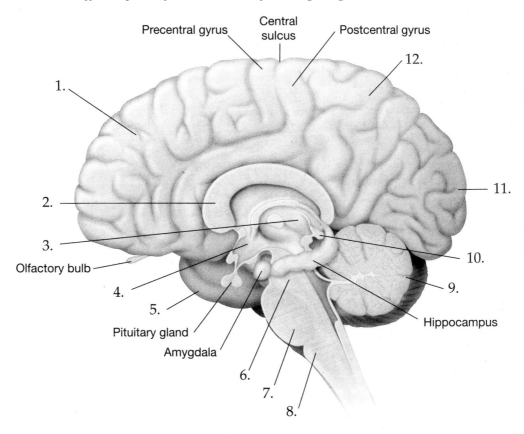

Precentral gyrus　Central sulcus　Postcentral gyrus

1.　2.　3.

Olfactory bulb　4.　5.

Pituitary gland　Amygdala　6.　7.　8.

12.　11.　10.　9.　Hippocampus

© Body Scientific International

1. Item 1:_____

2. Item 2:_____

3. Item 3:_____

4. Item 4:_____

5. Item 5:_____

6. Item 6:_____

7. Item 7:_____

8. Item 8:_____

9. Item 9:_____

10. Item 10:_____

11. Item 11:_____

12. Item 12:_____

Copyright Goodheart-Willcox Co., Inc.
May not be reproduced or posted to a publicly accessible website.

Terms Matching, Part 1

Instructions: *Match each of the following medical terms or abbreviations with the correct meaning.*

1. _____ condition caused by the degeneration of motor neurons in the spinal cord and in the brain's medulla and cortex

2. _____ condition generally discovered in newborns, in which a portion of the spinal cord and meninges protrudes through an opening in the spine

3. _____ condition characterized by unilateral facial paralysis

4. _____ condition caused by organic brain disease, which is characterized by memory loss, dysphonia, and difficulty performing routine tasks

5. _____ a brief stoppage of blood flow to a part of the brain

6. _____ inflammation of the gray matter of the spinal cord

7. _____ the sudden blockage of blood flow to the brain that results in death of brain tissue

8. _____ chronic, slow-progressing disease characterized by dyskinesia, dystaxia, paresthesia, and muscle weakness

A. ALS

B. Bell's palsy

C. CVA

D. dementia

E. MS

F. myelomeningocele

G. polio

H. TIA

Terms Matching, Part 2

Instructions: *Match each of the following medical terms or abbreviations with the correct meaning.*

1. _____ condition in which neuromuscular communication is disrupted and the muscles become severely weakened

2. _____ a disruption of electrical activity in the brain characterized by violent muscle contractions and loss of consciousness

3. _____ a state of confusion, agitation, and disorientation, usually accompanied by hallucinations

4. _____ a condition that occurs at or before birth, which affects movement and muscle tone

5. _____ the generalized term that describes the neurological disorder in which cells in the brain do not function correctly, causing seizures

6. _____ accumulation of CSF in the ventricles of the brain, which results in cephalomegaly and may cause brain damage

7. _____ abnormal, localized dilation of a blood vessel in the cerebrum

8. _____ a condition in which a newborn baby's meninges protrude through an opening of the skull or spinal cord

9. _____ a TBI resulting from a blow to the head or severe shaking of the head and upper body

10. _____ inflammation of multiple peripheral nerves, causing progressive muscle weakness. Usually occurs during or after recovery from an infectious disease

A. cerebral aneurysm

B. CP

C. concussion

D. delirium

E. epilepsy

F. GB syndrome

G. MG

H. hydrocephalus

I. meningocele

J. grand mal seizure

Copyright Goodheart-Willcox Co., Inc.
May not be reproduced or posted to a publicly accessible website.

CHAPTER 11 | The Special Senses

Activity A   Understanding Word Parts

Word Parts Matching, Part 1

Instructions: *Match each of the following word parts with the correct meaning.*

1. _____ droop; sag; prolapse; protrude
2. _____ ear condition
3. _____ disease
4. _____ to turn
5. _____ smell condition
6. _____ not; without
7. _____ outward
8. _____ inflammation
9. _____ hearing
10. _____ tumor; mass

A. exo-
B. -cusis
C. -itis
D. -oma
E. -ptosis
F. -tropia
G. -osmia
H. a-
I. -pathy
J. -otia

Word Parts Matching, Part 2

Instructions: *Match each of the following word parts with the correct meaning.*

1. _____ gray
2. _____ auditory tube; fallopian tube
3. _____ pupil
4. _____ eye
5. _____ double
6. _____ night
7. _____ light
8. _____ eardrum
9. _____ eyelid
10. _____ darkness

A. blephar/o
B. phot/o
C. dipl/o
D. nyct/o
E. core/o
F. glauc/o
G. salping/o
H. myring/o
I. scot/o
J. ocul/o

Copyright Goodheart-Willcox Co., Inc.
May not be reproduced or posted to a publicly accessible website.

Word Parts Matching, Part 3

Instructions: *Match each of the following word parts with the correct meaning.*

1. _____ pertaining to

2. _____ vision condition

3. _____ below; below normal; deficient

4. _____ process of measuring

5. _____ inward

6. _____ widened; enlarged

7. _____ old age

8. _____ lens of the eye

9. _____ tear

10. _____ taste

A. -ous

B. -metry

C. -opia

D. eso-

E. hypo-

F. presby/o

G. dacry/o

H. gustat/o

I. mydr/o

J. phak/o

Build the Medical Term

Instructions: *Use the prefixes, combining forms, and suffixes listed on pages 317–318 of your textbook to build the medical term that corresponds to each of the following definitions.*

1. Word part: an-

   Definition: condition of having no smell sense

   Term: _____

2. Word part: audi/o

   Definition: process of measuring hearing

   Term: _____

3. Word part: -algia

   Definition: ear pain

   Term: _____

4. Word part: -tic

   Definition: pertaining to (making) smaller

   Term: _____

Medical Terms and Definitions

Instructions: *Break down each of the following medical terms into its word parts (prefix, root word, combining vowel, and suffix if used). Then define each term.*

1. dacryocystitis

   Breakdown: _____

   Define: _____

2. amblyopia

   Breakdown: _____

   Define: _____

Copyright Goodheart-Willcox Co., Inc.
May not be reproduced or posted to a publicly accessible website.

3. myringoplasty

Breakdown: _____

Define: _____

4. retinoscope

Breakdown: _____

Define: _____

5. otosclerosis

Breakdown: _____

Define: _____

6. lacrimal

Breakdown: _____

Define: _____

Copyright Goodheart-Willcox Co., Inc.
May not be reproduced or posted to a publicly accessible website.

Activity B   Interpreting Medical Records

Instructions: *Read the following medical record. Identify the meaning of the abbreviations that appear in bold and are listed after the record, and then answer the following question.*

Medical Record

<u>See Clearly Eye Clinic</u>
<u>Dr. Ken U. Seamy</u>
Patient Name: Jose Ramirez
Date of Exam: April 3, 20XX
Medical Record No.: R3456

CC: Pt c/o difficulty with nighttime driving. Pt states, "I see halos around the lights when I try to drive after dusk." Pt states that this has restricted his activity, and that he must leave work early to avoid driving at night.

HPI: 62 y/o Hispanic male presents to clinic with c/o decreased **VA**, both distance and close up. He also states that his vision seems more "dull and cloudy" than normal. He first noticed symptoms about six months ago, and the visual problems have worsened since then. Pt currently does not wear glasses, but he states that he is "afraid that I am going to have to start wearing them because when I read the newspaper the words are blurry."

PMH: HTN controlled with diet and medication.

SH: Hx of smoking, but Pt states he quit about five years ago when he experienced an episode of **angina** and was **Dx** with **CAD**.

OH: Retired from the Army. Currently works as supervisor for a building construction company.

Current Medications: **OTC** multivitamins, fish oil. Prescription medications include lisinopril 20 **mg b.i.d.,** Lipitor 20 mg once a day.

PE: BP: 136/78. **PERRLA**, brows symmetrical, lashes intact, conjunctiva pink, no discharge noted, sclera white. VA 20/40 on **Snellen chart**. VA 20/30 with corrective lenses. VA 20/60 with glare test. **Bilateral** nuclear sclerotic cataracts noted.

Plan: Bilateral **phaco** with IOL (intraocular lens) implants. Schedule **O.D.** first, and then plan for second procedure on **O.S.** two weeks after that. Inform Pt that he will be able to return to work two days **postop**, but he should not lift anything over 10 pounds and needs to restrict outdoor exposure from two days **preop** to two weeks postop.

Medications to Be Dispensed:

Gaifloxacin ophthalmic solution: 4 **gtts q.i.d.** O.D. two days preop until two weeks postop

Ketoralac NSAID solution: 1 gtt every day two days preop until two weeks postop

Prednisolone ophthalmic solution: 1 gtt **t.i.d.** two days preop until one week postop
Repeat this order for O.S.

1. CC: _____

2. Pt: _____

3. c/o: _____

4. HPI: _____

5. VA: _____

6. PMH: _____

7. HTN: _____

8. SH: _____

9. Hx: _____

10. angina: _____

Copyright Goodheart-Willcox Co., Inc.
May not be reproduced or posted to a publicly accessible website.

11. Dx: _____

12. CAD: _____

13. OH: _____

14. OTC: _____

15. mg: _____

16. b.i.d.: _____

17. PE: _____

18. BP: _____

19. PERRLA: _____

20. Snellen chart: _____

21. Bilateral: _____

22. phaco: _____

23. O.D.: _____

24. O.S.: _____

25. postop: _____

26. preop: _____

27. gtts: _____

28. q.i.d.: _____

29. t.i.d.: _____

30. Which medical term describes the visual condition that this patient experiences when he is reading the newspaper?

_____

Copyright Goodheart-Willcox Co., Inc.
May not be reproduced or posted to a publicly accessible website.

Activity C   Comprehending Anatomy and Physiology Terminology

Definitions

Instructions: *Use pages 317–318 and the glossary in the back of your textbook to define the following terms.*

1. accommodation: _____

2. blind spot: _____

3. visual acuity: _____

4. pinna: _____

5. umami: _____

Review

Instructions: *Answer the following questions.*

1. What is the general function of the eyes, ears, nose, tongue, and skin—collectively known as the *specialized sense organs*?

   _____

2. Which term describes the "white of the eye"?

   _____

3. What is the purpose of the cornea?

   _____

4. Describe the ciliary muscle's function.

   _____

5. What substance is located in the front chamber of the eyeball?

   _____

6. What substance is located in the back chamber of the eyeball?

   _____

7. Which structures convert the images we see into nerve impulses?

   _____

8. Which structures allow us to see in color?

   _____

9. What is another term for the second cranial nerve?

   _____

10. Which term describes the area on the retina that produces the sharpest vision?

    _____

11. Which structure produces and excretes tears?

    _____

Copyright Goodheart-Willcox Co., Inc.
May not be reproduced or posted to a publicly accessible website.

12. When someone is crying, why might he or she experience a salty taste?

_____

13. What is the purpose of cerumen?

_____

Ear Identification

Instructions: *Label the different parts of the ear in the following image.*

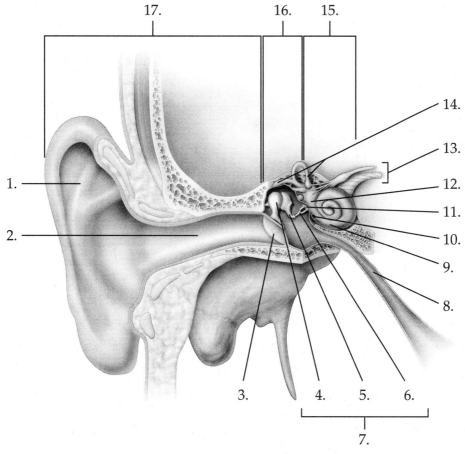

© *Body Scientific International*

1. Item 1:_____   10. Item 10:_____

2. Item 2:_____   11. Item 11:_____

3. Item 3:_____   12. Item 12:_____

4. Item 4:_____   13. Item 13:_____

5. Item 5:_____   14. Item 14:_____

6. Item 6:_____   15. Item 15:_____

7. Item 7:_____   16. Item 16:_____

8. Item 8:_____   17. Item 17:_____

9. Item 9:_____

Copyright Goodheart-Willcox Co., Inc.
May not be reproduced or posted to a publicly accessible website.

Activity D Understanding Terms Related to Diseases and Conditions

Matching

Instructions: *Match each of the following terms, which are related to conditions of the eye, to the correct meaning.*

1. _____ condition in which the eyelid turns inward

2. _____ misalignment of the eyes in which one or both eyes turn inward

3. _____ abnormal curvature of the cornea

4. _____ repetitive, usually involuntary eye movement

5. _____ clouding of the lens

6. _____ condition in which one or both eyes turn outward

7. _____ separation of the retina from its blood supply

8. _____ inflammation of an eyelid gland

9. _____ damage to the retina due to diabetes mellitus

10. _____ the presence of specks or lines in the field of vision

A. exotropia

B. retinal detachment

C. hordeolum

D. cataract

E. vitreous floaters

F. entropion

G. astigmatism

H. esotropia

I. diabetic retinopathy

J. nystagmus

Disease Identification

Instructions: *Identify the term that corresponds to each disease or condition described below.*

1. a fungal infection of the ear: _____

2. a ringing or buzzing sensation in the ears: _____

3. an impaired sense of taste: _____

4. a noncancerous tumor of the auditory nerve: _____

5. a disorder of the inner ear that results in vertigo: _____

6. a disease of the nerves: _____

7. hearing loss resulting from inadequate sound-wave conduction from the outer ear to bones of the middle ear:

_____

8. a condition characterized by a weakened sense of smell: _____

9. a condition, seen commonly in children, in which the middle ear becomes inflamed: _____

10. the condition in which the bones of the middle ear become hardened: _____

Copyright Goodheart-Willcox Co., Inc.
May not be reproduced or posted to a publicly accessible website.

Matching

Instructions: *Match each of the following medical terms with the correct synonym.*

1. _____ anosmia

2. _____ otomycosis

3. _____ myopia

4. _____ amblyopia

5. _____ otalgia

6. _____ cerumen

7. _____ hyperopia

8. _____ strabismus

9. _____ ophthalmodynia

10. _____ diplopia

A. double vision

B. earache

C. farsightedness

D. swimmer's ear

E. eye pain

F. earwax

G. crossed eyes

H. lazy eye

I. absence of smell

J. nearsightedness

Copyright Goodheart-Willcox Co., Inc.
May not be reproduced or posted to a publicly accessible website.

Activity E   Analyzing Diagnostic- and Treatment-Related Terms

Medical Terms and Definitions

Instructions: *Break down each of the following medical terms into its word parts (prefix, root word, combining vowel, and suffix if used). Then define each term.*

1. audiometry

   Breakdown: _____

   Define: _____

2. graphesthesia

   Breakdown: _____

   Define: _____

3. photocoagulation

   Breakdown: _____

   Define: _____

4. myringotomy

   Breakdown: _____

   Define: _____

Medical Scenarios

Instructions: *Read the following scenarios and answer the question in each one.*

1. Jason has applied for a job with the police department. He must pass a physical exam before he can start work. One part of the exam is a test that assesses his visual clarity using a Snellen chart. What is the name of this test?

   _____

   _____

2. Another part of Jason's testing includes a series of neurological exams that evaluates five kinds of responses to identify problems with the CNS or PNS. What is the name of these tests?

   _____

   _____

3. Peter Turner is an audiologist whose assignment is to evaluate workers at an offshore oil rig for hearing problems. He knows that he will need a specific instrument to inspect the workers' external auditory canals and tympanic membranes. Which instrument is this, and for which test is it used?

   _____

   _____

Copyright Goodheart-Willcox Co., Inc.
May not be reproduced or posted to a publicly accessible website.

4. Peter will also assess each worker's ability to detect sounds of different pitches. What equipment does he need for this test?

_____

_____

5. Peter is also expecting to perform a test that will assess the reactivity of the tympanic membrane to pressure changes. What is the name of this test, and which instrument does it require?

_____

_____

6. Laura is an RN in a busy HEENT specialist office. She is reviewing the patient roster for the day so that she can prepare exam rooms for the two doctors with whom she works. The first patient of the day is a 3 y/o with recurrent otitis media, otalgia, and hypertrophy of the tonsils and adenoids. Laura knows the doctor will need to perform a visual examination of the patient's ears. What piece of equipment does Laura need to have available in this patient's exam room?

_____

_____

7. When Laura reviewed the chart for the 3 y/o patient, she noticed that the child has been taking medication to prevent a bacterial infection of the middle ear. What is this medication's classification?

_____

_____

8. When the doctor evaluates this patient, she decides that surgery is necessary to treat the condition. The doctor recommends a tonsillectomy and an adenoidectomy. She also recommends a procedure in which a surgical incision is made into the eardrum and a pressure-equalizing tube is placed in the tympanic membrane. What is the name of this procedure?

_____

_____

9. The next patient is a 6 y/o boy who suffered from sensorineural hearing loss at birth. He had surgery three weeks ago to have an electronic device that will restore his hearing surgically implanted in the inner ear. What is the name of this procedure?

_____

_____

10. Dr. Westmoreland, OD, is starting a new practice in her hometown. What kind of specialist is Dr. Westmoreland?

_____

_____

11. While Dr. Westmoreland is unpacking her new equipment, she examines plates that will be used to test her patients for color blindness. In which test will these plates be used?

_____

_____

12. Dr. Westmoreland opens another box and finds the equipment she will use to examine the interior of her patients' eyes. What is the name of this test?

_____

_____

13. Next, she finds the equipment that is used to examine the front chamber of the eye with microscopic magnification. What is the name of this test?

_____

_____

14. There is also a box filled with pamphlets that contain information about surgery that will restore vision for those with cataracts. What is the name of this surgery?

_____

_____

15. Dr. Reyes is an ophthalmologist who specializes in emergency cases. He receives a call from the ER about the victim of a gunshot wound to the face. The left side of the victim's face was affected, and the eye is unable to be saved. Which surgery would Dr. Reyes perform to remove the affected eyeball?

_____

_____

16. Later that day, Dr. Reyes receives a call from the ER concerning a patient who was admitted with c/o flashing lights and a shadow that obstructed his vision. Dr. Reyes knows that these symptoms are caused by retinal detachment. This condition requires immediate treatment or it will result in blindness. Which surgery is used to treat this condition?

_____

_____

Copyright Goodheart-Willcox Co., Inc.
May not be reproduced or posted to a publicly accessible website.

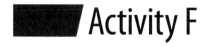 **Activity F**   Preparing for Your Future
in Healthcare

Defining Word Parts

Instructions: *Use the information on pages 317–318 of your textbook to define the following word parts.*

1. acoust/o: _____

2. audi/o: _____

3. blephar/o: _____

4. cochle/o: _____

5. opt/o: _____

6. phac/o: _____

7. presby/o: _____

8. -cusis: _____

9. -opia: _____

10. -otia: _____

Defining Medical Terms

Instructions: *Use a regular or medical dictionary, the Glossary/Index in the back of your textbook, and your own words to define the following terms.*

1. cochlear implant: _____

2. hyperopia: _____

3. myopia: _____

4. phacoemulsification: _____

5. presbycusis: _____

6. presbyopia: _____

7. vestibulocochlear nerve: _____

Identifying Healthcare Professionals

Instructions: *Identify the appropriate healthcare professional (optometrist, ophthalmologist, audiologist) that matches each of the following descriptions or tasks. You will use each profession more than once.*

1. requires a degree from a medical school: _____

2. treats patients with eye-related conditions: _____

3. can perform surgery: _____

4. may test newborns' hearing: _____

5. can dispense contact lenses: _____

6. treats patients with hearing-related conditions: _____

7. treats children: _____

8. can dispense hearing aids: _____

Copyright Goodheart-Willcox Co., Inc.
May not be reproduced or posted to a publicly accessible website.

Chapter 11 Practice Test

Definitions

Instructions: *Using the word parts on pages 317–318 of your textbook, identify the medical term that corresponds to each of the following definitions.*

1. inflammation of the eyelid:_____

2. disease of the retina: _____

3. "fear of," or sensitivity to, light: _____

4. hardening of the eardrum:_____

Medical Terms and Definitions

Instructions: *Break down each of the following medical terms into its word parts (prefix, root word, combining vowel, and suffix if used). Then define each term.*

1. aphakia

   Breakdown: _____

   Define:_____

2. keratotomy

   Breakdown: _____

   Define:_____

3. oculomycosis

   Breakdown: _____

   Define:_____

4. dacryocystocele

   Breakdown: _____

   Define:_____

5. retinoplasty

   Breakdown: _____

   Define:_____

6. mydriasis

   Breakdown: _____

   Define:_____

Review

Instructions: *Answer the following questions.*

1. Which five structures are generally considered organs of the special senses?

   _____

   _____

Copyright Goodheart-Willcox Co., Inc.
May not be reproduced or posted to a publicly accessible website.

2. Which four structures protect the eyeball?

_____

_____

3. What substance gives the eye its shape?

_____

4. Which structures allow for peripheral vision?

_____

5. At what age do a person's lacrimal glands start producing tears?

_____

6. Which glands produce earwax?

_____

7. What is the term for the hammer-shaped bone in the middle ear?

_____

8. Which term describes the cells in the nose that allow a person to smell?

_____

9. What is the medical term for chewing?

_____

10. Where are the sensory receptors for touch located?

_____

_____

Identifying Terms

Instructions: *Identify the term that corresponds to each disease, condition, test, or procedure described below.*

1. During a routine eye exam, an OD discovers that his patient has abnormally high intraocular pressure that has caused damage to the retina. Which term describes this condition?

_____

2. The doctor examines another patient who has a defective curvature of the cornea. What is this condition called?

_____

3. The next patient the doctor examines has a swollen, red eyelid gland that is filled with pus. Which term describes this condition?

_____

4. The first afternoon patient is scheduled for an eye test that will measure the area within which objects are seen when the eyes are in a fixed position. What is the name of this test?

_____

5. An ophthalmologist examines a patient who has been having difficulty with her vision, especially at night. The doctor notices that the patient's left lens is clouded. What diagnosis would the doctor write in this patient's chart?

_____

Copyright Goodheart-Willcox Co., Inc.
May not be reproduced or posted to a publicly accessible website.

6. A medical assistant escorts a patient into the exam room. This patient is walking unsteadily and has to put her hands on the wall to prevent herself from falling. She states that she feels like the room is spinning. What term does the MA write in the patient's chart to describe her complaint?

_____

7. When the doctor examines this patient, he determines that her condition is caused by a disorder of the inner ear. Which term will the doctor use to describe this patient's condition?

_____

8. The next patient that the MA puts in the room has nasal congestion and rhinorrhea. He complains of being unable to taste anything. What term would the MA use to describe this condition?

_____

9. This same patient also complains of ear pain. What is the medical term for this condition?

_____

10. An Air Force flight surgeon is performing neurological testing of the pilots on his base. One of the tests that he performs requires pilots to close their eyes and identify an object that is placed in their hand. This test is repeated with a different object in the other hand. What is the name of this test?

_____

Copyright Goodheart-Willcox Co., Inc.
May not be reproduced or posted to a publicly accessible website.

CHAPTER 12 The Endocrine System

Activity A   Understanding Word Parts

Word Parts Matching, Part 1

Instructions: *Match each of the following word parts with the correct meaning.*

1. _____ urination; condition of urine
2. _____ below; below normal; deficient
3. _____ hormone
4. _____ like; resembling
5. _____ many; much
6. _____ swelling; fluid retention
7. _____ above; above normal; excessive
8. _____ to analyze
9. _____ thirst
10. _____ enlargement

A. -edema
B. -megaly
C. -dipsia
D. -assay
E. hypo-
F. poly-
G. -tropin
H. -oid
I. -uria
J. hyper-

Word Parts Matching, Part 2

Instructions: *Match each of the following word parts with the correct meaning.*

1. _____ sex glands
2. _____ female; woman
3. _____ X-rays
4. _____ cortex
5. _____ secrete
6. _____ breast
7. _____ potassium
8. _____ mucus
9. _____ ketone
10. _____ calcium

A. mast/o
B. myx/o
C. crin/o
D. kal/i
E. calc/o
F. ket/o
G. gonad/o
H. radi/o
I. gynec/o
J. cortic/o

Copyright Goodheart-Willcox Co., Inc.
May not be reproduced or posted to a publicly accessible website.

Build the Medical Term

Instructions: *Use the combining forms and suffixes listed on pages 352–353 of your textbook to build the medical term that corresponds to each of the following definitions.*

1. Word part: glyc/o

   Definition: condition of sugar in the urine

   Term: _____

2. Word part: tox/i

   Definition: condition of poison in the blood

   Term: _____

3. Word part: thyroid/o

   Definition: inflammation of the thyroid gland

   Term: _____

4. Word part: -ic

   Definition: pertaining to the eye

   Term: _____

5. Word part: thyr/o

   Definition: enlargement of the thyroid gland

   Term: _____

Medical Terms and Definitions

Instructions: *Break down each of the following medical terms into its word parts (prefix, root word, combining vowel, and suffix if used). Then define each term.*

1. polydipsia

   Breakdown: _____

   Define: _____

2. hypoinsulinemia

   Breakdown: _____

   Define: _____

3. gigantism

   Breakdown: _____

   Define: _____

4. adrenocorticotropin

   Breakdown: _____

   Define: _____

5. hyperglycemia

   Breakdown: _____

   Define: _____

Copyright Goodheart-Willcox Co., Inc.

May not be reproduced or posted to a publicly accessible website.

◢ Activity B   Interpreting Medical Records

Instructions: *Read the following medical record. Identify the meaning of the abbreviations that appear in bold and are listed after the record, and then answer the following questions.*

Medical Record

A-1C Endocrine Clinic

Dr. B. Shaw, **ATT PHY**

Patient Name: John Davidson

Date of Birth: 12/4/19XX

Medical Record No.: DJ543

Subjective Data: A 54 y/o male presents to a clinic with c/o fatigue, tingling, and numbness in the **distal** lower extremities; **polydipsia**; **polyuria**; and **polyphagia**. Pt states that these symptoms began about a year ago after he changed jobs. At his current job, he spends most of the day at a desk.

PE: well-developed male; wt: 230 lbs; **P**: 72 **bpm**; **BP**: 144/92; **FBS**: 145 **mg/dL**; **GTT** results: 210 mmol/L

Dx: hyperglycemia, NIDDM, obesity, borderline **HTN**

Tx: Start pt on Metformin 500 **mg b.i.d.**

Dispense home glucose monitor and check blood sugar levels **q.i.d.**, **a.c.**, and **h.s.**

Consult with **CDE** for diet counseling and disease management

Refer to **CFT** for exercise plan

Set up pt for **EKG** to R/O **CAD**

Pt to return to clinic every week to recheck BP and FBS

Follow up with Dr. Shaw in 3 months

1. ATT PHY: _____

2. distal: _____

3. polydipsia: _____

4. polyuria: _____

5. polyphagia: _____

6. P: _____

7. bpm: _____

8. BP: _____

9. FBS: _____

10. mg/dl: _____

11. GTT: _____

12. Dx: _____

13. hyperglycemia: _____

14. NIDDM: _____

15. obesity: _____

16. HTN: _____

Copyright Goodheart-Willcox Co., Inc.

May not be reproduced or posted to a publicly accessible website.

17. Tx:_____

18. mg: _____

19. b.i.d.: _____

20. q.i.d.: _____

21. a.c.: _____

22. h.s.: _____

23. Consult:_____

24. CDE: _____

25. CFT: _____

26. EKG:_____

27. CAD:_____

28. When is Mr. Davidson supposed to check his blood sugar levels at home?

_____

_____

29. Which complaint indicates that Mr. Davidson may be developing complications related to his diagnosis?

_____

_____

30. Which medical term describes the complaint referenced in the previous question?

_____

_____

Copyright Goodheart-Willcox Co., Inc.
May not be reproduced or posted to a publicly accessible website.

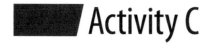 ## Activity C   Comprehending Anatomy and Physiology Terminology

Definitions

Instructions: *Use a regular or medical dictionary, the Glossary/Index in the back of your textbook, and your own words to define the following terms.*

1. circadian rhythm

   _____

   _____

2. cortex

   _____

   _____

3. gland

   _____

   _____

4. medulla

   _____

   _____

5. tropins

   _____

   _____

Review

Instructions: *Answer the following questions.*

1. List the primary organs and glands of the endocrine system.

   _____

2. Which gland controls all the other endocrine glands?

   _____

3. Which gland is important in regulating the body's "sleep-and-waking" cycle?

   _____

4. Which two glands are located in the throat?

   _____

5. Which two hormones, secreted by the thyroid and the parathyroid glands, counteract each other?

   _____

6. Which cells secrete the hormone that helps lower blood sugar?

   _____

Copyright Goodheart-Willcox Co., Inc.
May not be reproduced or posted to a publicly accessible website.

7. Which cells secrete the hormone that helps raise blood sugar?

_____

8. What is the medical term for sex cells?

_____

9. Which term describes the female gonads?

_____

10. What causes a male's voice to develop a deeper sound?

_____

Terms Matching

Instructions: *Match each of the following hormones with the correct function.*

1. _____ helps maintain pregnancy

2. _____ stimulates the deposit of calcium into the bones and lowers blood calcium levels

3. _____ stimulates uterine contractions during childbirth and the release of milk in females who are breastfeeding

4. _____ triggers the body's fight-or-flight response

5. _____ regulates blood pressure, electrolyte levels, and fluid volume

6. _____ controls metabolism and body temperature

7. _____ stimulates ovulation and controls menstruation

8. _____ regulates the absorption of glucose into blood cells

9. _____ stimulates the thyroid gland and helps regulate thyroid function

10. _____ regulates blood glucose levels and helps metabolize carbohydrates, proteins, and fats

A. aldosterone

B. calcitonin

C. cortisol

D. epinephrine

E. insulin

F. LH

G. oxytocin

H. progesterone

I. TSH

J. T_3

Copyright Goodheart-Willcox Co., Inc.
May not be reproduced or posted to a publicly accessible website.

Name _____

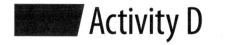 Activity D   Understanding Terms Related
to Diseases and Conditions

Medical Terms and Definitions

Instructions: *Break down each of the following medical terms into its word parts (prefix, root word, combining vowel, and suffix if used). Then define each term.*

1. acidosis

    Breakdown: _____

    Define: _____

    _____

    _____

2. adenocarcinoma

    Breakdown: _____

    Define: _____

    _____

    _____

3. gynecomastia

    Breakdown: _____

    Define: _____

    _____

    _____

4. hyperparathyroidism

    Breakdown: _____

    Define: _____

    _____

    _____

5. hyponatremia

    Breakdown: _____

    Define: _____

    _____

    _____

Copyright Goodheart-Willcox Co., Inc.
May not be reproduced or posted to a publicly accessible website.

Interpreting Medical Scenarios

Instructions: *Imagine that you are job-shadowing Ruth, an RN who is the head office nurse for Dr. White, an endocrinologist. Ruth is reviewing the patient roster for the day. Read the following scenarios and answer the question in each one.*

1. The first patient of the morning is Joe. According to the new patient information sheet, Joe is a former body builder. While reviewing the referral from Joe's primary care physician, you notice she has requested an evaluation by Dr. White because Joe has recently gained a lot of weight. Joe's listed weight is 20 percent more than the average for his age, sex, build, and height. Which term describes this condition?

_____

2. On the lab reports provided by his PCP, Joe's cortisol levels are well above what is considered normal for him. Ruth calls Joe back into the room so that she can take his vital signs. Ruth weighs Joe, and you notice that his ankles and feet are swollen. Which medical term describes this condition?

_____

3. You also notice that Joe has several bruises on his legs and arms. Ruth takes Joe's blood pressure and records the result in his chart as 150/100. You remember from class that anything above 120/80 is considered higher than normal. What term would you expect Ruth to use to describe Joe's blood pressure reading?

_____

4. Dr. White comes into the room to examine Joe. During the interview, Joe tells Dr. White that he used anabolic steroids for several years. He states that he has not used any steroids in more than six months. Joe complains of feeling weak and not having the energy he had when using steroids. What do you think Dr. White's diagnosis for Joe will be?

_____

5. The next appointment is an urgent evaluation for Andrea, a 35-year-old female who was admitted to the ER last night with extreme anxiety and muscle spasms. Lab work performed in the ER shows that Andrea's blood calcium levels are well below normal. Which term describes the muscle condition Andrea was experiencing while in the ER?

_____

6. Ruth escorts Andrea into an exam room. During the interview, Andrea tells Ruth that she suffered a fracture of her distal fibula three months ago. Ruth reviews the X-ray and notices that the bone seems to have healed without any complications. However, Andrea's orthopedic specialist ordered a bone density test, and the results showed significant bone loss, especially for Andrea's age. Dr. White reviews the lab work from the ER and notices that Andrea's PTH level is elevated. What do you think is Andrea's diagnosis?

_____

7. Jean is a 54-year-old female with complaints of unexpected weight loss and abnormal anxiety. She was evaluated by her PCP, who referred her to Dr. White. While Ruth is weighing the patient, you notice that Jean's face looks peculiar. You look closer and notice that Jean's eyes are bulging slightly and appear larger than you would expect. Which term describes this condition?

_____

8. Dr. White palpates Jean's neck and tells Ruth to document hypertrophy of the thyroid gland. What does this mean?

_____

_____

9. While reviewing the lab reports on Jean's chart, you notice that her T_3 and T_4 levels are elevated. Which term describes this condition?

_____

Copyright Goodheart-Willcox Co., Inc.
May not be reproduced or posted to a publicly accessible website.

10. Dr. White explains to Jean that she has an autoimmune condition that has caused her thyroid gland to become overactive. Which medical term describes this diagnosis?

_____

11. Andy is a 19 y/o male who has had DM since childhood. Now, as a college student, he is not managing his condition as well as he did when he was at home. Andy requires insulin injections q.i.d. and sometimes he "forgets" to check his blood sugar. Which term describes Andy's condition?

_____

12. Dr. White tells Andy that he is going to have to treat his hyperglycemia or he will have complications. What does the term *hyperglycemia* mean?

_____

_____

_____

13. You remember learning about a condition in which the retina of the eye can be damaged as a complication of DM. Which term describes this condition?

_____

14. Dr. White explains to Andy that he may also start experiencing pain and weakness, especially in his hands and feet. Which term describes this condition?

_____

15. Andy tells Dr. White that he recently spent three days in the hospital. Andy said the doctor told him that he had an acute episode of diabetic ketoacidosis. Andy asked Dr. White to explain this condition to him. What would you expect Dr. White to tell Andy?

_____

_____

_____

Copyright Goodheart-Willcox Co., Inc.
May not be reproduced or posted to a publicly accessible website.

Activity E   Analyzing Diagnostic- and Treatment-Related Terms

Matching

Instructions: *Match each of the following terms with the correct meaning.*

1. _____ test that measures the amounts of thyroxine in the blood by testing for levels of triiodothyronine

2. _____ test in which a camera is used to record the accumulation of a radioactive chemical as it moves into the thyroid

3. _____ test that requires a patient to collect urine for 24 hours

4. _____ test that determines the amount of protein-bound iodine in the blood

5. _____ test considered to be the most accurate for measuring thyroid activity

6. _____ test that measures the amount of triiodothyronine in the blood

7. _____ test that measures the amount of human chorionic gonadotropin in the blood

8. _____ test that uses sound waves to produce a visual image of the endocrine gland in the throat

9. _____ test that measures the amount of thyroxine in the blood

10. _____ test that determines whether a person is pregnant

A. catecholamines test

B. quantitative HCG test

C. TSH test

D. thyroid ultrasound

E. T_3RU test

F. qualitative HCG test

G. T_4 test

H. PBI test

I. T_3 test

J. thyroid scan

Disease or Condition Identification

Instructions: *Identify the term that corresponds to each of the following described procedures or treatments.*

1. What might be a treatment option for a 10-year-old male with a diagnosis of dwarfism?

_____

_____

2. What is a possible treatment option for a 53-year-old female with Graves' disease and exophthalmos?

_____

_____

3. Which drug treatment should be used for a 6-year-old female with a diagnosis of IDDM?

_____

_____

Copyright Goodheart-Willcox Co., Inc.
May not be reproduced or posted to a publicly accessible website.

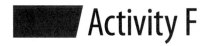 Activity F   Preparing for Your Future
in Healthcare

Define Abbreviations

Instructions: *Define each of the following abbreviations.*

1. CDE: _____

2. DI: _____

3. FBS: _____

4. IDDM: _____

5. NIDDM: _____

6. SIADH: _____

Definitions

Instructions: *Use a regular or medical dictionary, the Glossary/Index in the back of your textbook, and your own words to define the following terms.*

1. hormones: _____

2. infertility: _____

3. menopause: _____

4. phlebotomy: _____

Healthcare Professional Identification

Instructions: *Identify the appropriate healthcare professional (nutritionist, endocrinologist, certified diabetes educator, phlebotomist) that matches the following descriptions or tasks. You will use each profession more than once.*

1. assists people with diet planning: _____

2. requires a degree from a medical school: _____

3. may work in a school: _____

4. requires some college coursework: _____

5. may work in a blood bank: _____

6. may educate people with IDDM on how to administer their medications: _____

7. generally receives on-the-job training during coursework: _____

8. may treat people experiencing infertility: _____

9. will prepare blood to be sent to the laboratory: _____

10. requires a state license: _____

Copyright Goodheart-Willcox Co., Inc.
May not be reproduced or posted to a publicly accessible website.

Chapter 12 Practice Test

Identification

Instructions: *Identify the term that corresponds to each disease or condition described below.*

1. condition of deficient glucose in the blood: _____

2. condition of excessive potassium in the blood: _____

3. the surgical removal of a breast: _____

4. condition of excessive urination: _____

Medical Terms and Definitions

Instructions: *Break down each of the following medical terms into its word parts (prefix, root word, combining vowel, and suffix if used). Then define each term.*

1. retinoblastoma

   Breakdown: _____

   Define: _____

2. panhypopituitarism

   Breakdown: _____

   Define: _____

3. thyrotoxicosis

   Breakdown: _____

   Define: _____

Matching

Instructions: *Match each of the following terms with the correct meaning.*

1. _____ condition of being smaller or shorter than normal

2. _____ disease caused by insufficient secretion of cortisol and sometimes aldosterone

3. _____ tumor of the adrenal gland that secretes excess epinephrine and norepinephrine

4. _____ disease caused by inadequate secretion of ADH by the posterior pituitary gland

5. _____ a malignant tumor of any gland or mucus-secreting organ

6. _____ condition in which the body produces acidic ketone bodies as a result of high blood glucose levels

7. _____ general term that describes any condition in which the body experiences an increase in the acidity of the blood, body fluids, or tissues

8. _____ disease in which insulin production is normal, but the body cannot use the insulin efficiently

9. _____ condition in which a male develops abnormally large mammary glands

A. adenocarcinoma

B. type 2 diabetes mellitus

C. pheochromocytoma

D. diabetic ketoacidosis

E. Addison's disease

F. acidosis

G. diabetes insipidus

H. dwarfism

I. gynecomastia

Copyright Goodheart-Willcox Co., Inc.
May not be reproduced or posted to a publicly accessible website.

Hormone Definition

Instructions: *Define each of the following abbreviations for hormones, and then indicate which gland in the endocrine system secretes the hormone.*

1. ACTH

   Meaning: _____

   Gland: _____

2. ADH

   Meaning: _____

   Gland: _____

3. CRH

   Meaning: _____

   Gland: _____

4. FSH

   Meaning: _____

   Gland: _____

5. GH

   Meaning: _____

   Gland: _____

6. GHIH

   Meaning: _____

   Gland: _____

7. GHRH

   Meaning: _____

   Gland: _____

8. GnRH

   Meaning: _____

   Gland: _____

9. MSH

   Meaning: _____

   Gland: _____

10. PTH

    Meaning: _____

    Gland: _____

11. T_3

    Meaning: _____

    Gland: _____

Copyright Goodheart-Willcox Co., Inc.
May not be reproduced or posted to a publicly accessible website.

12. T$_4$

Meaning: _____

Gland: _____

13. TRH

Meaning: _____

Gland: _____

14. TSH

Meaning: _____

Gland: _____

Copyright Goodheart-Willcox Co., Inc.
May not be reproduced or posted to a publicly accessible website.

CHAPTER 13 The Urinary System

Activity A   Understanding Word Parts

Word Parts Matching, Part 1

Instructions: *Match each of the following word parts with the correct meaning.*

1. _____ hernia; swelling; protrusion
2. _____ urination; condition of urine
3. _____ breakdown; separation; loosening
4. _____ substance that forms
5. _____ crushing
6. _____ between
7. _____ hardening; thickening
8. _____ surgical fixation
9. _____ not; without
10. _____ abnormal condition

A. inter-
B. -poietin
C. -cele
D. -iasis
E. -sclerosis
F. -lysis
G. -uria
H. -tripsy
I. an-
J. -pexy

Word Parts Matching, Part 2

Instructions: *Match each of the following word parts with the correct meaning.*

1. _____ cyst; fluid sac; bladder
2. _____ meatus
3. _____ nitrogen
4. _____ bacteria
5. _____ night
6. _____ kidney
7. _____ urinary bladder
8. _____ scanty
9. _____ calyx
10. _____ renal pelvis

A. olig/o
B. cali/o
C. pyel/o
D. azot/o
E. meat/o
F. nephr/o
G. cyst/o
H. noct/o
I. bacteri/o
J. vesic/o

Copyright Goodheart-Willcox Co., Inc.
May not be reproduced or posted to a publicly accessible website.

Build the Medical Term

Instructions: *Use the combining forms and suffixes listed on pages 382–383 of your textbook to build the medical term that corresponds to each of the following definitions.*

1. Word part: -ar

   Definition: pertaining to the glomerulus

   Term: _____

2. Word part: nephr/o

   Definition: hardening or thickening of the kidney

   Term: _____

3. Word part: cyst/o

   Definition: inflammation of the bladder

   Term: _____

Medical Terms and Definitions

Instructions: *Break down each of the following medical terms into its word parts (prefix, root word, combining vowel, and suffix if used). Then define each term.*

1. cystoscopy

   Breakdown: _____

   Define: _____

2. dialysis

   Breakdown: _____

   Define: _____

3. nephrectomy

   Breakdown: _____

   Define: _____

4. genitourinary

   Breakdown: _____

   Define: _____

5. ureterostenosis

   Breakdown: _____

   Define: _____

6. cystolithotomy

   Breakdown: _____

   Define: _____

7. nephropexy

   Breakdown: _____

   Define: _____

Copyright Goodheart-Willcox Co., Inc.
May not be reproduced or posted to a publicly accessible website.

8. hydronephrosis

   Breakdown: _____

   Define: _____

9. anuria

   Breakdown: _____

   Define: _____

10. hematuria

    Breakdown: _____

    Define: _____

11. urethrospasm

    Breakdown: _____

    Define: _____

12. retroperitoneal

    Breakdown: _____

    Define: _____

Copyright Goodheart-Willcox Co., Inc.

May not be reproduced or posted to a publicly accessible website.

Activity B   Interpreting Medical Records

Medical Record Interpretation

Instructions: *Read the following medical record. Define the abbreviations and medical terms called out in the record. Then answer the questions that follow.*

Medical Record

Kidney Wellness Center

Dr. Amy Murphy

Patient Name: Mary Sanders

Date of Birth: 3-12-19XX

Medical Record No.: 56347

Date of Exam: 5-3-20XX

Subjective Data: **Pt** is a 32 **y/o** female who had a normal vaginal delivery of her third child nine months ago. There were no complications with the pregnancy, labor, or delivery. She has **c/o incontinence** since the birth. Pt has tried exercise but symptoms have not improved. She must wear a pad at all times. She has stopped running because she is worried about having an accident before she can reach a bathroom. Because she has not been able to exercise as much as she did before having her last child, she has gained about 20 lbs. Pt was evaluated by **OB/GYN** and her uterus was found to be **WNL**. Pt was referred to urology for evaluation and recommendation of **tx** options. Pt is a **NS**.

Objective Data: **wt**: 160 lbs; **ht**: 65"; **P**: 76; **R**: 14; **T**: 97.6°; **BP**: 120/64

HEENT: WNL

CV Hx: not significant

GU *Hx*: Three pregnancies, three live births, all delivered vaginally without complications. No recent history of **UTI** or **nephrolithiasis**. Pt reports that she uses about four pads a day, depending on her activity level. Pt states that leakage increases with sneezing or laughing. Pt denies **dysuria**, **hematuria**, and **polyuria**. No changes in medication noted. Pt has no history of abdominal surgery.

PE: **Cystocele** noted with vaginal examination.

Assessment: Grade 1 cystocele. **Internal urethral sphincter** deficiency.

Recommendation: Collect urine via straight in-and-out **CATH** for **UA**.

Schedule Pt for **VCUG**.

Refer Pt to **PT** for recommendation and teaching exercises to strengthen pelvic floor muscles.

1. Pt: _____

2. y/o: _____

3. c/o: _____

4. incontinence: _____

_____

_____

5. OB/GYN: _____

6. WNL: _____

7. tx: _____

8. NS: _____

9. wt: _____

Copyright Goodheart-Willcox Co., Inc.
May not be reproduced or posted to a publicly accessible website.

10. ht: _____

11. P: _____

12. R: _____

13. T: _____

14. BP: _____

15. HEENT: _____

16. CV: _____

17. Hx: _____

18. GU: _____

19. UTI: _____

20. nephrolithiasis: _____

_____

_____

21. dysuria: _____

_____

_____

22. hematuria: _____

_____

_____

23. polyuria: _____

_____

_____

24. PE: _____

25. cystocele: _____

_____

_____

26. Internal urethral sphincter: _____

_____

_____

27. CATH: _____

28. UA: _____

29. VCUG: _____

30. PT: _____

Copyright Goodheart-Willcox Co., Inc.
May not be reproduced or posted to a publicly accessible website.

31. Why do you think this patient is experiencing incontinence?

_____

_____

_____

_____

Test Identification

Instructions: *Imagine that you work as a student intern in the laboratory at UMC hospital. You have just received the samples for several doctor's offices. Which test is indicated by each of the following abbreviations?*

1. BUN: _____

2. CBC: _____

3. Hct: _____

4. Hgb: _____

5. GFR: _____

6. pH: _____

7. FBS: _____

8. PKU: _____

9. sp gr: _____

Copyright Goodheart-Willcox Co., Inc.
May not be reproduced or posted to a publicly accessible website.

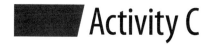 **Activity C   Comprehending Anatomy and Physiology Terminology**

Definitions

Instructions: *Use a regular or medical dictionary, the Glossary/Index in the back of your textbook, and your own words to define the following terms.*

1. filtration: _____

   _____

2. excretion: _____

   _____

3. ions: _____

   _____

4. homeostasis: _____

   _____

5. urinary tract: _____

   _____

6. electrolytes: _____

   _____

7. urination: _____

   _____

8. nephron: _____

   _____

9. filtrate: _____

   _____

10. urea: _____

   _____

Word Part Definitions

Instructions: *Using the information on pages 382–383, define the following word parts.*

1. cyst/o: _____

2. glomerul/o: _____

3. peritone/o: _____

4. pyel/o: _____

5. ureter/o: _____

6. retro-: _____

Copyright Goodheart-Willcox Co., Inc.
May not be reproduced or posted to a publicly accessible website.

Review

Instructions: *Answer the following questions.*

1. What are the four main functions of the urinary system?

   _____

   _____

2. Which hormone produced by the kidneys stimulates hematopoiesis?

   _____

3. List the three ways in which the kidneys help the body maintain homeostasis.

   _____

   _____

4. Which term describes the area behind the membranous lining of the abdominopelvic cavity?

   _____

5. Which three terms are used to describe the discharge of urine from the bladder?

   _____

Kidney Labeling

Instructions: *Label the parts of the kidney in the following image.*

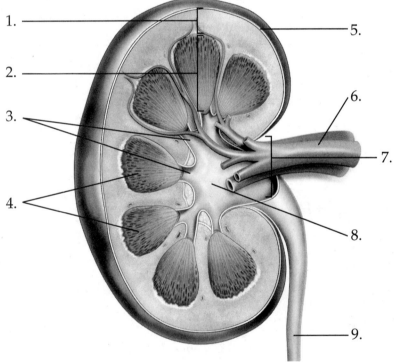

© *Body Scientific International*

1. Item 1:_____   6. Item 6:_____

2. Item 2:_____   7. Item 7:_____

3. Item 3:_____   8. Item 8:_____

4. Item 4:_____   9. Item 9:_____

5. Item 5:_____

Copyright Goodheart-Willcox Co., Inc.
May not be reproduced or posted to a publicly accessible website.

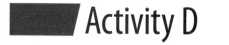 **Activity D   Understanding Terms Related to Diseases and Conditions**

Match Medical Terms

Instructions: *Match each of the following medical terms with the correct meaning.*

1. _____ the presence of sugars in the urine

2. _____ difficult or painful urination

3. _____ loss of voluntary control over the discharge of urine from the bladder

4. _____ an inability to completely empty the bladder

5. _____ absence of urine production

6. _____ bed wetting

7. _____ involuntary discharge of urine

8. _____ condition in which a small amount of urine is produced

9. _____ the sudden, urgent need to urinate

10. _____ abnormal increase in the production of urine

A. urinary incontinence

B. oliguria

C. urinary retention

D. diuresis

E. glycosuria

F. anuria

G. enuresis

H. urinary urgency

I. dysuria

J. nocturnal enuresis

Disease or Condition Identification

Instructions: *Identify the term that corresponds to each disease or condition described.*

1. inflammation of the lining of the renal pelvis and the kidney: _____

2. inflammation of the bladder: _____

3. inflammation of the glomeruli in the kidney: _____

4. chronic inflammation of the bladder wall: _____

5. condition of stones in the kidney: _____

6. condition of stones in the bladder: _____

7. condition in which the bladder protrudes through a weakened place in the vaginal wall:

_____

8. condition in which an abnormal opening forms between the bladder and vagina: _____

9. cancerous tumor of the kidney in a 65 y/o male: _____

10. cancerous tumor of the kidney in a 5 y/o male: _____

11. condition of the kidney in which damage or disease causes impaired filtration: _____

12. condition in which the arteriole walls of the kidneys become narrowed and thickened:

_____

13. condition characterized by the development of fluid-filled sacs within the kidney, leading to nephromegaly:

_____

Copyright Goodheart-Willcox Co., Inc.
May not be reproduced or posted to a publicly accessible website.

Activity E   Analyzing Diagnostic- and Treatment-Related Terms

UA Result Identification

Instructions: *Imagine that you are a certified medical assistant (CMA) working in a busy specialists' office. The providers in this office include Dr. Cindy Pate, a urologist; Dr. Sam Greene, a nephrologist; and Dr. Tamera Lyons, an endocrinologist. One of your most common tasks is to perform an in-office UA on almost every patient. It is important for you to know the normal results for a UA. Identify what you would expect to be normal for each of the following observations that you make when performing this test.*

1. color: _____

_____

2. pH: _____

_____

3. protein: _____

_____

4. glucose: _____

_____

5. ketones: _____

_____

6. occult hematuria: _____

_____

7. leukocytes: _____

_____

8. nitrates: _____

_____

9. bilirubin: _____

_____

Medical Scenarios

Instructions: *Read the following scenarios and answer the questions.*

1. In addition to the UA, you routinely perform a test that requires you to spin a urine sample in a special machine to separate the urine's solids from its liquid. What is the name of the machine that you would use for this test?

_____

2. You also educate your patients about a test that requires them to collect their urine for a 24-hour period and take it to the lab, where it will be tested along with a sample of blood to determine how well the glomeruli in the kidneys are functioning. What is the name of this test?

_____

3. You routinely draw blood and send it to the lab to measure the amount of waste products in the blood. What is the name of this test?

_____

Copyright Goodheart-Willcox Co., Inc.
May not be reproduced or posted to a publicly accessible website.

4. You review the patient list for the day to make sure you have all of the test results ready for the doctors to review before they see their patients. The first chart you check for Dr. Pate is a patient who had an X-ray test in which the kidneys, ureters, and bladder were viewed using a contrast agent. What is the name of this test?

_____

5. Dr. Greene has a patient named Bob Gomez who has recently had a shunt placed in his left forearm so that he can undergo treatments that will filter his blood through a machine and return cleansed blood to his system. What is the name for this treatment?

_____

6. Mr. Gomez had a test performed to evaluate the blood vessels of his kidney. This test uses a contrast medium and a camera that records the flow of blood. What is the name of this test?

_____

7. Mr. Gomez had this test performed because he will soon be added to a list of people waiting to receive a donor kidney. What procedure will Mr. Gomez undergo if he receives a donor kidney?

_____

8. Dr. Lyons is seeing a patient named Mrs. Wilma Robinson. Mrs. Robinson has lived with IDDM for 25 years. She has also been dealing with a chronic UTI for the past six months. She has been taking medication to treat this condition, but the infection keeps coming back. Which classification of medication should she be taking to treat this infection?

_____

9. Dr. Lyons has consulted with Dr. Pate concerning Mrs. Robinson. They decided that Dr. Pate would perform a visual examination of the urinary bladder to identify any abnormalities. What is the name of this test?

_____

10. While reviewing Mrs. Robinson's chart, you discover that she received treatment for a bladder stone three years ago. This treatment used high-energy shock waves to break up the stone. What is the name of this treatment?

_____

11. After this treatment, Mrs. Robinson went home with a flexible tube placed in her bladder. The tube exited through her urethra so that her bladder would not fill up with urine. What is the name of this procedure?

_____

12. Jerry McDaniel is a patient of Dr. Pate's who recently had a kidney removed due to polycystic kidney disease. What is the name of this surgery?

_____

13. Jerry has developed some lower extremity edema. To treat this problem, Dr. Pate is going to put Jerry on a trial of a medication that will increase his urine output. What is the classification of this medication?

_____

14. Dr. Pate wants to schedule Jerry for a test that will determine how his remaining kidney is functioning. This test is an X-ray visualization of the renal pelvis, ureters, and bladder using a contrast medium. What is the name of this test?

_____

15. Dr. Greene's next patient is Tyler, a six-year-old male who was diagnosed with Wilms tumor. This diagnosis came after a procedure in which a small amount of the tumor's tissue was removed from the kidney using a hollow needle to be evaluated by a pathologist. What is the name of this procedure?

_____

16. Dr. Greene wants Tyler to undergo a radiographic test in which images of the kidney and abdominal area are taken from multiple angles using a contrast medium and analyzed by a computer. What is the name of this procedure?

_____

Copyright Goodheart-Willcox Co., Inc.
May not be reproduced or posted to a publicly accessible website.

Activity F   Preparing for Your Future in Healthcare

Word Part Definitions

Instructions: *Using the information on pages 382–383, define the following word parts.*

1. iatr/o:_____

2. -ic:_____

3. -logist:_____

4. nephr/o:_____

5. onc/o:_____

6. ur/o:_____

Definitions

Instructions: *Use a regular or medical dictionary, the Glossary/Index in the back of your textbook, and your own words to define the following terms.*

1. dialysis:_____

2. nephrologist:_____

3. oncologist:_____

4. urologist:_____

Healthcare Professional Descriptions

Instructions: *Identify the appropriate healthcare professional (dialysis technician, urologist, case management nurse) that matches each of the following descriptions. You will use each profession more than once.*

1. I must receive orders from a doctor or nurse before I can begin my treatments:_____

2. I graduated from nursing school:_____

3. I have my own private practice:_____

4. I operate equipment designed to eliminate toxins from the blood of patients whose kidneys are not functioning properly:_____

5. I may visit a patient at home:_____

6. I must pass a test given by BONENT before I can work:_____

7. I graduated from medical school:_____

8. I can only work in a hospital or outpatient clinic setting:_____

9. I coordinate a patient's care with other members of the healthcare team:_____

10. I can treat bladder cancer:_____

11. I graduated from a technical school:_____

12. I can receive a certification from ACMA:_____

13. I can perform surgery for male sterilization:_____

14. I can receive certification from NNCO:_____

15. It is important that I understand the cost of a patient's healthcare needs:_____

Copyright Goodheart-Willcox Co., Inc.
May not be reproduced or posted to a publicly accessible website.

▰▰▰ Chapter 13 Practice Test

Word Part Definitions

Instructions: *Using the word parts on pages 382–383 of your textbook, identify the medical term that corresponds to each of the following definitions.*

1. condition of scanty urination: _____

2. condition of much urination: _____

3. condition of pus in the urine: _____

4. surgical repair of the ureter: _____

5. inflammation of the peritoneum: _____

Medical Terms and Definitions

Instructions: *Break down each of the following medical terms into its word parts (prefix, root word, combining vowel, and suffix if used). Then define each term.*

1. nephromegaly

   Breakdown: _____

   Define: _____

2. ureterolithiasis

   Breakdown: _____

   Define: _____

3. cystorrhaphy

   Breakdown: _____

   Define: _____

4. vesicotomy

   Breakdown: _____

   Define: _____

5. azotemia

   Breakdown: _____

   Define: _____

Review

Instructions: *Answer the following questions.*

1. Define the term *filtration*.

   _____

   _____

   _____

2. What is the function of calcitriol, a hormone produced by the kidneys?

   _____

   _____

3. List the three regions of the kidney.

   _____

Copyright Goodheart-Willcox Co., Inc.
May not be reproduced or posted to a publicly accessible website.

4. Where are the functional units of the kidney located?

_____

5. In which part of the nephron does reabsorption take place?

_____

6. What are the five major components of urine?

_____

_____

7. Which term describes the depression in a kidney that serves as a passageway for blood vessels, lymphatic vessels, and nerves?

_____

8. Approximately how much volume can the urinary bladder hold before the brain is notified that it is time to be emptied?

_____

9. How long is the female urethra?

_____

Disease or Condition Identification

Instructions: *Identify the term that corresponds to each disease or condition described below.*

1. scanty urination: _____

2. no urine production: _____

3. presence of blood in the urine: _____

4. difficult or painful urination: _____

5. involuntary discharge of urine at night: _____

Diagnosis Identification

Instructions: *Identify the correct diagnosis for each patient described below.*

1. 35 y/o male with symptoms of hyperglycemia, polydipsia, polyuria, and deficiency of insulin in the blood:

_____

2. 45 y/o female with multiple cysts in the kidney accompanied by nephromegaly:

_____

3. 28 y/o male with severe lower back pain and positive X-ray for renal calculi:

_____

Test or Treatment Identification

Instructions: *Identify the correct test or treatment described in each situation below.*

1. treatment in which high-energy shock waves are used to attempt to break up renal calculi:

_____

2. an examination of the urine to test for abnormal elements:

_____

3. removal of the kidney:

_____

Copyright Goodheart-Willcox Co., Inc.
May not be reproduced or posted to a publicly accessible website.

CHAPTER 14 — The Male Reproductive System

Activity A   Understanding Word Parts

Word Parts Matching, Part 1

Instructions: *Match each of the following word parts with the correct meaning.*

1. _____ below; below normal; deficient
2. _____ formation
3. _____ across
4. _____ pertaining to breakdown or destruction
5. _____ flow; excessive discharge
6. _____ condition of growth or development
7. _____ around; surrounding
8. _____ surgical opening
9. _____ enlargement
10. _____ surgical fixation

A. -pexy
B. -megaly
C. -trophy
D. -genesis
E. -rrhea
F. hypo-
G. trans-
H. -lytic
I. peri-
J. -stomy

Word Parts Matching, Part 2

Instructions: *Match each of the following word parts with the correct meaning.*

1. _____ female; woman
2. _____ male
3. _____ vessel; duct
4. _____ hidden
5. _____ testis
6. _____ glans penis
7. _____ animal; life
8. _____ tumor
9. _____ sexual contact
10. _____ breast

A. vas/o
B. gyn/o
C. mast/o
D. andr/o
E. zo/o
F. crypt/o
G. onc/o
H. balan/o
I. vener/o
J. orchi/o

Copyright Goodheart-Willcox Co., Inc.
May not be reproduced or posted to a publicly accessible website.

Build the Medical Term

Instructions: *Use the combining forms listed on pages 414–415 of your textbook to build the medical term that corresponds to each of the following definitions.*

1. Word part: spermat/o

   Definition: formation of sperm

   Term: _____

2. Word part: orchi/o

   Definition: surgical fixation of a testicle

   Term: _____

3. Word part: sperm/o

   Definition: pertaining to the destruction of sperm

   Term: _____

Medical Terms and Definitions

Instructions: *Break down each of the following medical terms into its word parts (prefix, root word, combining vowel, and suffix if used). Then define each term.*

1. azoospermia

   Breakdown: _____

   Define: _____

2. anorchism

   Breakdown: _____

   Define: _____

3. transrectal

   Breakdown: _____

   Define: _____

4. prostatovesiculitis

   Breakdown: _____

   Define: _____

5. electrocautery

   Breakdown: _____

   Define: _____

6. andropathy

   Breakdown: _____

   Define: _____

7. balanoplasty

   Breakdown: _____

   Define: _____

Copyright Goodheart-Willcox Co., Inc.
May not be reproduced or posted to a publicly accessible website.

▮▮▮▮ Activity B   Interpreting Medical Records

Instructions: *Read the medical record that follows. Identify the meaning of the abbreviations that appear in bold and are listed after the record. Then answer the questions that follow.*

Medical Record

Sunshine Valley Urology Clinic
Dr. Gary Thomas, MD
3100 N. Happy Trails Drive, Ste 250
Sunnyville, CO 12345

PMH: 52 y/o male with Hx of **NIDDM** for 15 years. Pt manages condition with oral medications. **FBS** ranges from 80 to 138 **mg/dl** for the past three months. Pt has not complained of changes in **VA** and states that he is evaluated annually by his **ophthalmologist**. Pt has started noticing numbness and tingling in his toes, especially when his blood sugar is greater than 120 mg/dl. Pt has recently experienced difficulty achieving and maintaining an erection during sexual activity. Pt was evaluated by PCP and **endocrinologist**, and then referred to the urology department for evaluation and Tx.

SH: Pt is a **NS** and denies frequent alcohol consumption, although he admits to having an occasional beer with his friends about once a month. Pt denies recreational drug use.

OH: Pt is a high school math teacher.

FH: Pt's father had a **Dx** of **DM** for 40 years and passed away at age 70 of a **MI**. Pt's mother has a Dx of **AD** and is living in a nursing home. Pt has two brothers who are living—one, age 56, has a Dx of **CAD** and **CHF**, and the other, age 58, suffers from **COPD**. Pt had a sister who passed away at age 35 of **SLE**.

Psychosocial: Pt has been married to same spouse for 24 years. They have spent the past 10 summers serving on various overseas church mission trips. Pt and his spouse have three adult children together. One child is in the military and is currently overseas. Their middle child is married and has two children. Their youngest child is in college. Pt admits that the burden of caring for his aging mother, having a child in college, and having another child overseas in the military has caused a mental and financial burden, but he states, "I think I am handling it well." Pt does admit that his inability to achieve an erection has caused him some anxiety, but he states that his spouse is very understanding.

PE: ht: 72 inches; wt: 191.2 pounds

HEENT: deferred

CV: P: 74 bpm; **BP**: 152/92; heart sounds: WNL

Dorsal pedal pulses slightly less predominant than radial and carotid pulses, bilaterally. Normal rate and rhythm of pulses.

GU: Circumcised penis noted without discharge or abnormalities. Scrotal sac appears WNL. **DRE** reveals a normally sized prostate gland. Pt denies **dysuria**, **nocturia**, or **hematuria**. Recent ultrasound of genitals reveals a mild decrease in blood flow to the penis.

Lab: **CBC** is WNL

Kidney and liver function is WNL

Testosterone, **LH**, **FSH**, prolactin, T_3, T_4, and **TSH** are all WNL

Cholesterol: 215 mg/dl

Impression: Dx of **ED** secondary to DM

Plan: Recommend a low-fat/low-cholesterol diet. Refer back to PCP for evaluation of **HTN**. Trial of sildenafil with 50 mg **p.o.** daily, to be taken about 30 minutes to 4 h prior to sexual activity. Pharmacist to educate pt on side effects and precautions involved with this medication. Pt should follow up in four months, or sooner if indicated.

1. PMH: _____

2. NIDDM: _____

3. FBS: _____

4. mg/dl: _____

5. VA: _____

6. ophthalmologist: _____

7. endocrinologist: _____

8. SH: _____

9. NS: _____

10. FH: _____

11. Dx: _____

12. DM: _____

13. MI: _____

14. AD: _____

15. CAD: _____

16. CHF: _____

17. COPD: _____

18. SLE: _____

19. CV: _____

20. BP: _____

21. DRE: _____

22. dysuria: _____

23. nocturia: _____

24. hematuria: _____

25. CBC: _____

26. LH: _____

27. FSH: _____

28. T_3: _____

29. T_4: _____

30. TSH: _____

31. ED: _____

32. HTN: _____

33. p.o.: _____

34. Describe where you would find each of the following pulses.

　A. dorsal pedal pulse: _____

　B. radial pulse: _____

　C. carotid pulse: _____

35. What did the urologist determine in his physical examination that caused him to refer this patient back to his PCP?

_____

Copyright Goodheart-Willcox Co., Inc.
May not be reproduced or posted to a publicly accessible website.

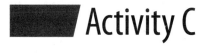 **Activity C** **Comprehending Anatomy and Physiology Terminology**

Definitions

Instructions: *Use a regular or medical dictionary, the Glossary/Index in the back of your textbook, and your own words to define the following terms.*

1. sperm: _____

2. spermatogenesis:_____

3. semen: _____

4. puberty:_____

5. ejaculation: _____

Word Part Definitions

Instructions: *Using the information on pages 414–415 of your textbook, define the following word parts.*

1. balan/o: _____

2. orchi/o: _____

3. semin/o: _____

4. test/o: _____

5. vas/o:_____

Testis and Epididymis Labeling

Instructions: *Label the parts of the testis and epididymis in the following image.*

1. Item 1:_____

2. Item 2:_____

3. Item 3:_____

4. Item 4:_____

5. Item 5:_____

6. Item 6:_____

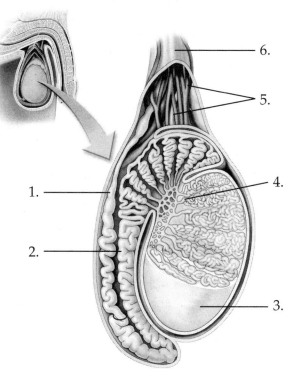

© *Body Scientific International*

Copyright Goodheart-Willcox Co., Inc.
May not be reproduced or posted to a publicly accessible website.

Review

Instructions: *Answer the following questions.*

1. What is the main purpose of the male reproductive system?

   _____

2. Which term describes the fertilization of the ovum?

   _____

3. How are gametes different from other body cells?

   _____

4. What are the two external components of the male reproductive system?

   _____

5. Where do sperm mature until they are ready for fertilization?

   _____

6. Why is it important that the testes are located outside of the abdominal cavity?

   _____

7. Which hormone stimulates the testes to produce testosterone?

   _____

8. What is the purpose of the flagellum?

   _____

9. What is the main purpose of semen?

   _____

10. What is the main purpose of the prostate gland?

    _____

11. Which gland helps lubricate body surfaces during sexual intercourse?

    _____

12. How does the penis become erect during sexual intercourse?

    _____

13. Which internal anatomical structure of the male reproductive system is also considered part of the urinary system?

    _____

Copyright Goodheart-Willcox Co., Inc.
May not be reproduced or posted to a publicly accessible website.

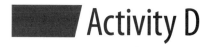 **Activity D** **Understanding Terms Related to Diseases and Conditions**

Determine the Term

Instructions: *Imagine that you are the radiologist at a children's hospital. You are reviewing the ultrasound results for a two-day old male patient. Determine the term for the patient's condition in each of the following situations.*

1. the right testicle has not descended into the scrotal sac: _____

2. the left testicle is surrounded by a fluid-filled sac: _____

3. an abnormal enlargement of the vein in the spermatic cord of the right testicle: _____

Instructions: *Imagine that you are a nurse practitioner at a health clinic. Determine the diagnosis in the following cases.*

1. a 23-year-old male comes into the clinic complaining of painful urination:

_____

2. another male patient has discharge of pus from the end of his penis:

_____

3. the shaft of another patient's penis has warts on it:

_____

4. another patient is experiencing sores on the mucous membranes in his mouth, a rash on his hands and feet, sore throat, fatigue, and hair loss:

_____

Physician Assistant Medical Scenarios

Instructions: *Imagine that you are a recent graduate who has been hired as a physician assistant at a rural health clinic that specializes in male health. Your first patient of the day is Mr. Johnston, a 58-year-old male. Read the following descriptions and answer the accompanying questions.*

1. Mr. Johnston has been complaining of having to urinate frequently. What is this condition called?

_____

2. Mr. Johnston also tells you that it is difficult for him to start urinating. He feels like he "needs to go," but then it takes him longer to empty his bladder than it used to take. Which term describes the inability to completely empty the bladder?

_____

3. You review Mr. Johnston's recent lab work and notice that his PSA is WNL. What does the PSA test measure?

_____

4. You perform a DRE. What is this procedure?

_____

5. You discover that Mr. Johnston's prostate gland is enlarged. What three medical terms can be used to describe this condition?

_____

Copyright Goodheart-Willcox Co., Inc.
May not be reproduced or posted to a publicly accessible website.

6. Why is Mr. Johnston having difficulty urinating?

_____

Medical Assistant Scenarios

Instructions: *Imagine that you are the medical assistant for Dr. Henrietta Haines, a reproductive endocrinologist who specializes in infertility. Read the following scenarios and answer the accompanying questions.*

1. Dr. Haines sees many patients who are struggling with infertility. To meet the definition of infertility, for how long must a couple have practiced unprotected sex and been unable to achieve pregnancy?

_____

2. When Dr. Haines interviews a couple, she will ask them about their own personal health histories, including the diagnosis and treatment of STIs and any other medical conditions. Which condition involves the abnormal location of the testis or testicles at birth and can affect fertility after puberty?

_____

3. Which medical term describes a problem with the spermatic cord that can affect a male's fertility?

_____

4. Lab tests are routinely performed on a male's sperm to identify any potential causes of infertility. Which condition is characterized by a low sperm count?

_____

Patient Education Specialist Scenarios

Instructions: *Imagine that you are a registered nurse working in an oncology department as a patient education specialist. Your supervisor has asked you to develop a seminar for males. You know that it is important to present information that is relevant to the audience. Answer the following questions, which address important health issues for males.*

1. There are specific types of cancer that affect males. What is the most common type of cancer in males older than 50 years of age?

_____

2. You decide to also emphasize the importance of TSE. What type of cancer is determined during this procedure?

_____

3. Accidents that occur during recreational sports may cause serious injury to the spermatic cord, which can cut off the blood supply to the testes. Which term describes this condition?

_____

Copyright Goodheart-Willcox Co., Inc.
May not be reproduced or posted to a publicly accessible website.

Name _____

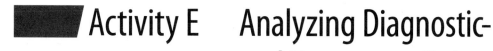 **Activity E   Analyzing Diagnostic- and Treatment-Related Terms**

Word Part Matching

Instructions: *Match each of the following word parts with the correct meaning.*

1. _____ pertaining to

2. _____ rectum

3. _____ around

4. _____ to cut

5. _____ across

6. _____ surgical fixation

7. _____ sexual contact

8. _____ surgical opening

9. _____ heat; burn

10. _____ process; state; condition

A. trans-

B. vener/o

C. cauter/o

D. rect/o

E. -ion

F. -pexy

G. -al

H. circum-

I. -stomy

J. cis/o

Review

Instructions: *Answer the following questions.*

1. A patient named Mr. Lee presents with c/o dysuria and polyuria. He has been diagnosed with BPH, and his PSA is WNL. What does this mean?

   _____

   _____

2. To help diagnose Mr. Lee's condition, the doctor orders a test that delivers sound waves to the pelvic area. What is the name of this test?

   _____

3. The urologist recommends a TRUS for Mr. Lee. Describe this procedure.

   _____

4. It is determined that Mr. Lee does not have prostate cancer. However, since Mr. Lee is experiencing dysuria and polyuria, the urologist recommends a procedure in which a section of the prostate gland is removed through the urethra. What is the name of this procedure?

   _____

5. During preop instructions, the doctor tells Mr. Lee that he will have a Foley catheter placed into his bladder during the procedure, and that he will possibly go home with it for a few days. What is this device?

   _____

6. After the procedure, the recovery room nurse monitors Mr. Lee for hematuria. Describe this condition.

   _____

Copyright Goodheart-Willcox Co., Inc.
May not be reproduced or posted to a publicly accessible website.

7. Which surgical procedure is often performed on newborn males to remove the foreskin of the penis?

_____

8. The removal of the foreskin is recommended to reduce the risk of which three conditions?

_____

_____

9. Which surgical procedure is performed to secure an undescended testis into the scrotal sac?

_____

10. What is the general term for a surgical procedure that can involve electrocautery or cryosurgery, and which is often performed to remove a cancerous area of the prostate gland?

_____

11. Which two terms describe the procedure in which needles are inserted into the prostate gland to direct radio waves that aid in shrinking the prostate gland?

_____

12. Which surgical procedure involves the removal of the entire prostate gland, as well as the seminal vesicles and surrounding tissue?

_____

13. What is the purpose of TFT testing?

_____

_____

14. Which surgical procedure, when performed on a male, results in sterilization?

_____

15. Which term describes the reversal of the procedure described in the previous question?

_____

Copyright Goodheart-Willcox Co., Inc.
May not be reproduced or posted to a publicly accessible website.

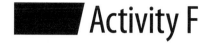 **Activity F**   **Preparing for Your Future in Healthcare**

Instructions: *Imagine that you are the manager of a large hospital's human resources department. You have been asked to revise the organization's employee job descriptions. Using the information on page 432 of your textbook, list the job tasks and educational requirements for each of the following healthcare professionals.*

Surgical Technician

1. Typical Tasks:

_____

_____

_____

_____

2. Educational Requirements:

_____

_____

Pharmacist

1. Typical Tasks:

_____

_____

_____

_____

2. Educational Requirements:

_____

_____

Oncologist

1. Typical Tasks:

_____

_____

_____

_____

2. Educational Requirements:

_____

_____

Copyright Goodheart-Willcox Co., Inc.
May not be reproduced or posted to a publicly accessible website.

Chapter 14 Practice Test

Definitions

Instructions: *Using the word parts on pages 414–415 of your textbook, identify the medical term that corresponds to each of the following definitions.*

1. excision of the vas deferens (vessel; duct): _____

2. inflammation of the epididymis: _____

3. inflammation of the glans penis: _____

4. excessive flow from the prostate gland: _____

Medical Terms and Definitions

Instructions: *Break down each of the following medical terms into its word parts (prefix, root word, combining vowel, and suffix if used). Then define each term.*

1. phimosis

   Breakdown: _____

   Define: _____

2. gonorrhea

   Breakdown: _____

   Define: _____

3. varicocele

   Breakdown: _____

   Define: _____

4. hyperplasia

   Breakdown: _____

   Define: _____

5. orchiectomy

   Breakdown: _____

   Define: _____

6. transrectal

   Breakdown: _____

   Define: _____

Copyright Goodheart-Willcox Co., Inc.
May not be reproduced or posted to a publicly accessible website.

Review

Instructions: *Answer the following questions.*

1. In which structure does spermatogenesis take place?

   _____

2. What is another name for sperm?

   _____

3. Which term describes a developing, fertilized ovum?

   _____

4. Which term describes the period of time in which secondary sexual characteristics become evident?

   _____

5. Are sperm cells larger or smaller than ovum cells?

   _____

6. Where are sperm stored until they are transported through the vas deferens?

   _____

Matching

Instructions: *Match each of the following diseases or conditions with the correct meaning.*

1. _____ condition of one or two undescended testicles
2. _____ infection of the skin and mucosa of the genitals caused by HSV
3. _____ benign prostatic hyperplasia (BPH)
4. _____ inflammation of the epididymis
5. _____ condition of an abnormally low sperm count
6. _____ stage of a chronic STI in which there may be no symptoms
7. _____ sexually transmitted infection (STI) caused by a parasite
8. _____ condition caused by the twisting of the spermatic cord
9. _____ inflammation of the prostate
10. _____ congenital absence of one or both testes

A. epididymitis
B. oligospermia
C. trichomoniasis
D. prostatomegaly
E. anorchia
F. cryptorchidism
G. latent syphilis
H. prostatitis
I. herpes genitalis
J. testicular torsion

Test Identification

Instructions: *Identify the term that corresponds to each test described below.*

1. involves palpation of the prostate to check for hypertrophy: _____

2. performed by a male to self-check for abnormalities of the testes: _____

3. measures the amount of sugar in the blood after a person has not eaten for at least 12 hours: _____

4. used to screen pregnant females for syphilis: _____

5. used to evaluate a male's fertility related to his semen: _____

6. involves the evaluation of the tissue of the prostate gland: _____

7. isolates and identifies bacteria that may be causing various infections: _____

Copyright Goodheart-Willcox Co., Inc.
May not be reproduced or posted to a publicly accessible website.

Treatment Identification

Instructions: *Identify the term that corresponds to each treatment described below.*

1. drugs used to treat impotence: _____

2. surgery to correct chronic phimosis:_____

3. surgery to correct cryptorchidism: _____

4. surgery to repair a varicocele:_____

5. surgery to treat testicular cancer which involves removal of a testis:_____

Copyright Goodheart-Willcox Co., Inc.
May not be reproduced or posted to a publicly accessible website.

CHAPTER 15 / The Female Reproductive System

▓▓▓ Activity A   Understanding Word Parts

Word Parts Matching, Part 1

Instructions: *Match each of the following word parts with the correct meaning.*

1. _____ new
2. _____ to bear (offspring)
3. _____ before
4. _____ beginning
5. _____ pregnant
6. _____ suture
7. _____ no; none
8. _____ state of pregnancy
9. _____ first
10. _____ childbirth

A. primi-
B. -arche
C. -gravida
D. nulli-
E. -partum
F. -rrhaphy
G. neo-
H. ante-
I. -para
J. -cyesis

Word Parts Matching, Part 2

Instructions: *Match each of the following word parts with the correct meaning.*

1. _____ milk
2. _____ ovary
3. _____ fallopian tube
4. _____ vagina
5. _____ breakdown; dissolve; loosen
6. _____ to bind; tie
7. _____ place; location; position
8. _____ vulva
9. _____ to enlarge or expand
10. _____ birth

A. nat/i
B. ly/o
C. ligat/o
D. oophor/o
E. lact/o
F. dilat/o
G. colp/o
H. episi/o
I. salping/o
J. top/o

Copyright Goodheart-Willcox Co., Inc.
May not be reproduced or posted to a publicly accessible website.

Build the Medical Term

Instructions: *Use the combining forms and suffixes listed on pages 438–439 of your textbook to build the medical term that corresponds to each of the following definitions.*

1. Word part: mast/o

   Definition: removal of a breast

   Term: _____

2. Word part: mamm/o

   Definition: process of recording a breast

   Term: _____

3. Word part: -ion

   Definition: process of binding or tying

   Term: _____

4. Word part: -cyesis

   Definition: state of a false pregnancy

   Term: _____

Medical Terms and Definitions

Instructions: *Break down each of the following medical terms into its word parts (prefix, root word, combining vowel, and suffix if used). Then define each term.*

1. hysterosalpingogram

   Breakdown: _____

   Define: _____

2. vulvovaginitis

   Breakdown: _____

   Define: _____

3. gynopathy

   Breakdown: _____

   Define: _____

4. hysteropexy

   Breakdown: _____

   Define: _____

5. oligomenorrhea

   Breakdown: _____

   Define: _____

6. salpingo-oophorectomy

   Breakdown: _____

   Define: _____

Copyright Goodheart-Willcox Co., Inc.
May not be reproduced or posted to a publicly accessible website.

◼ Activity B   Interpreting Medical Records

Instructions: *Read the medical record that follows. Identify the meaning of the abbreviations that appear in bold and are listed after the record. Then answer the questions that follow.*

Medical Record

<u>Morning Glory Women's Health Clinic</u>
Patient Name: Rose Williams
Date of Birth: 7-4-19XX
Medical Record No.: 35791
Date of Exam: 8-14-20XX

Subjective Data: Pt is a 48 y/o female with extensive **gynecology** hx. **Menarche** occurred at age 13. Episode of **TSS** occurred at age 17, requiring hospitalization for three weeks. Pt received Dx of **cervical dysplasia** at age 18. Tx with **conization**. Subsequent **Pap tests** have been **WNL**. Pt married at age 20. Husband passed away six months ago at age 49 of prostate cancer. Pt has not been sexually active for the past 4 years. Pt is gravida 4, para 2, **AB** 2. Obstetrical hx includes spontaneous AB x 2 at ages 23 and 24. **D&C** was performed after each miscarriage. At age 25, Pt had a normal vaginal delivery of a live male by **CNM**. At age 27, Pt had **CS** of a live female by **OB/GYN** due to **breech birth**. Pt started on **OCPs** after the delivery of her second child but stopped taking them at age 30 due to excessive wt gain and **HA**. Pt's husband had **vasectomy** performed. Pt began experiencing severe pelvic pain at age 32. Exploratory **laparotomy** performed and diagnosis of **ovarian cyst** and **endometriosis** confirmed. Symptoms subsided about six months after procedure. Pt had experienced normal periods after laparotomy, but in the past six years she has developed increasingly irregular periods, **dysmenorrhea**, **oligomenorrhea**, and breakthrough bleeding between periods. Recent pelvic ultrasound revealed **PCOS** and **uterine fibroid** tumors. Pt's mother and sister have both had hysterectomies due to uterine cancer.

Objective Data: wt: 185 lb; ht: 64"; P: 80 bpm; **R**: 15; **T**: 98.6°; BP: 136/78

PE: **HEENT**: **PERRLA**, no mass or **adenomegaly**. **Palpation** of thyroid glands showed no lesions. Excessive hair growth noted on lower jaw line, extending down onto neck.

CV: Heart rate and rhythm normal, good capillary refill of digits

GU: Abdomen palpated, no obvious lesions or abnormalities noted. Well-healed lower lateral incision noted. Visual exam of perineum reveals well-healed **episiotomy** scar. Internal pelvic examination reveals enlarged ovaries, R>L. Uterus is tender during palpation, approximately six weeks size.

Assessment: PCOS with **hirsutism** and uterine fibroids

Plan: **TAH-BSO**; refer to endocrinology for **HRT postop**

1. gynecology: _____

2. menarche: _____

3. TSS: _____

4. cervical dysplasia: _____

5. conization: _____

6. Pap tests: _____

7. WNL: _____

8. AB: _____

9. D&C: _____

10. CNM: _____

11. CS: _____

Copyright Goodheart-Willcox Co., Inc.
May not be reproduced or posted to a publicly accessible website.

12. OB/GYN: _____

13. breech birth: _____

14. OCPs: _____

15. HA: _____

16. vasectomy: _____

17. laparotomy: _____

18. ovarian cyst: _____

19. endometriosis: _____

20. dysmenorrhea: _____

21. oligomenorrhea: _____

22. PCOS: _____

23. uterine fibroids: _____

24. R: _____

25. T: _____

26. HEENT: _____

27. PERRLA: _____

28. adenomegaly: _____

29. palpation: _____

30. episiotomy: _____

31. hirsutism: _____

32. TAH-BSO: _____

33. HRT: _____

34. postop: _____

35. What was the probable cause of the patient's diagnosis and hospitalization at age 17?

    _____

36. What was the probable cause of the patient's diagnosis of cervical dysplasia at age 18?

    _____

37. How many times has Mrs. Williams been pregnant?

    _____

38. What might cause the doctor to suspect that Mrs. Williams has hirsutism?

    _____

39. Why does Mrs. Williams have a lower lateral incision on her abdomen?

    _____

40. Why does Mrs. Williams have an episiotomy scar on her perineum?

    _____

Copyright Goodheart-Willcox Co., Inc.
May not be reproduced or posted to a publicly accessible website.

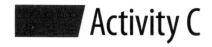 **Activity C** **Comprehending Anatomy and Physiology Terminology**

Term Identification

Instructions: *Identify the term that corresponds to each of the following descriptions.*

1. the female sex cell: _____

2. the structure in which a female sex cell matures: _____

3. the gland in the brain that facilitates function of the ovaries: _____

4. the two hormones secreted by the ovaries: _____

5. the phase of development in which the sexual organs mature: _____

6. the structures located on the ends of the fallopian tubes that help direct the ova: _____

7. the muscular contraction and relaxation that helps move the ovum to the uterus: _____

8. the top of the uterus: _____

9. the outermost layer of the uterus: _____

10. the area where pubic hair is located: _____

11. the female erectile tissue: _____

12. the ducts that carry breast milk to the nipples: _____

13. the darker-colored circle around the nipple of the breast: _____

Review

Instructions: *Answer the following questions.*

1. When is the fertilized ovum considered an embryo?

_____

_____

2. When is the embryo considered a fetus?

_____

3. What does the term *gestation* mean?

_____

4. What does the term *effacement* mean?

_____

5. What is the purpose of the labia?

_____

6. How is colostrum different from regular breast milk?

_____

Copyright Goodheart-Willcox Co., Inc.
May not be reproduced or posted to a publicly accessible website.

Developing Fetus Labeling

Instructions: *Label the different structures associated with a developing fetus in the following image.*

1. Item 1:_____

2. Item 2:_____

3. Item 3:_____

4. Item 4:_____

5. Item 5:_____

6. Item 6:_____

7. Item 7:_____

8. Item 8:_____ .

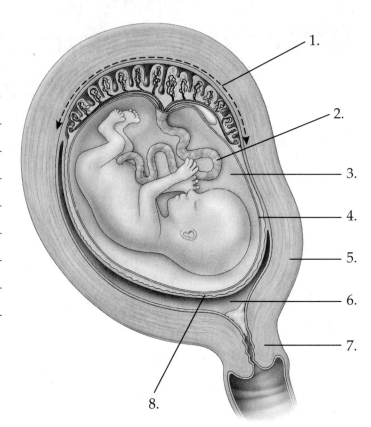

© *Body Scientific International*

Review

Instructions: *Answer the following questions.*

1. What is the typical length of a human's gestation period?

   _____

2. How is the first trimester defined?

   _____

3. How is the second trimester defined? the third?

   _____

   _____

4. What three major events occur during the first stage of labor?

   _____

5. In what position do most babies travel through the birth canal?

   _____

6. What occurs during the third stage of labor?

   _____

Copyright Goodheart-Willcox Co., Inc.
May not be reproduced or posted to a publicly accessible website.

Name _____

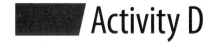 **Activity D** **Understanding Terms Related to Diseases and Conditions**

Registered Nurse Medical Scenarios

Instructions: *Imagine that you are a registered nurse for a large OB/GYN practice. You are reviewing the scheduled patients for the day so that you can prepare the rooms and necessary equipment for each appointment. Read each of the following scenarios and answer the accompanying questions.*

1. The first patient is Linda Overton, a 54 y/o G3 P3 AB0. Mrs. Overton has c/o dysuria, frequent UTIs, and incontinence. On her previous visit, Mrs. Overton was diagnosed with a hernia of the bladder that bulges through the anterior vaginal wall, and a hernia of the rectum that bulges through the posterior vaginal wall. During this appointment, the doctor will prepare Mrs. Overton for surgery. What are the two preop dx for this patient?

   _____

2. The next patient is Amber Gray, a 25 y/o G0 P0 who has been experiencing pelvic pain and cramping, and who has been unable to get pregnant. The doctor suspects that Amber has endometrial tissue that has developed outside of her uterus. The doctor is going to schedule her for an exploratory laparoscopy. What is this patient's preop dx?

   _____

3. You notice that Rosa Longoria is scheduled to come in. You remember talking to her several months ago when she called the office with c/o mastodynia. Last week, she had her routine mammogram, and the radiologist reported several fibrous tumors in both breasts, which did not appear to be cancerous. The radiologist recommended evaluation for possible treatment options. What is the preliminary diagnosis for Mrs. Longoria?

   _____

4. The last patient of the day is Rachel Edmondson, a 54 y/o G6 P5 AB0. She made the appointment because she feels like her "insides are falling out into her vagina." She also complains of difficulty with urination, incontinence, and chronic yeast infection. Which term describes Mrs. Edmondson's yeast infection?

   _____

5. You suspect that Mrs. Edmondson's uterus is displaced due to weakened ligaments that normally hold it in place. Which term describes this condition?

   _____

Nurse Practitioner Medical Scenarios

Instructions: *Imagine that you are a nurse practitioner at a prenatal clinic. Read the following scenarios and answer the accompanying questions.*

1. Trisha, a 16 y/o G2 P0 AB2 who is in for a follow-up on her recent Pap test, is in room one. She came to the clinic to get a prescription for birth control pills. Her Pap test came back positive for cervical dysplasia. When you explain this condition to Trisha, which virus will you say is the common cause?

   _____

2. How is this virus spread?

   _____

3. What is another uncomfortable condition that can be caused by this virus?

   _____

Copyright Goodheart-Willcox Co., Inc.
May not be reproduced or posted to a publicly accessible website.

4. If cervical dysplasia is not treated, which serious complication may occur?

_____

5. Nona, a 25 y/o G1 P1 AB0 who has been undergoing treatment for chlamydia, is in room two. Nona has been experiencing pelvic pain for several months now. What condition do you suspect Nona has?

_____

6. What is an additional complication of this condition that can affect the fallopian tubes and result in infertility?

_____

Medical Assistant Scenarios

Instructions: *Imagine that you are the medical assistant at a women's clinic. Read the following scenarios and answer the accompanying questions.*

1. The first patient you place in a room is Janice, a 25 y/o G5 P0 AB4 who is seeing the doctor for her six-week prenatal visit. Janice has a hx of spontaneous AB. Her first pregnancy ended at four weeks, her second ended at five weeks, and her third and fourth each ended at six weeks. Janice is very anxious about this visit. Her recent ultrasound showed the placenta was implanted at the lower end of the uterus. What is the medical term used to describe this condition?

_____

2. The next patient you place in a room is Chloe, a 35 y/o G1 P0 AB1. Chloe has been trying to get pregnant for 10 years and has experienced one spontaneous AB at five weeks gestation. Chloe wants to explore tx options for her infertility, but she is concerned because she had a friend whose zygote implanted in the fallopian tube, nearly resulting in death. What is the medical term for her friend's condition?

_____

3. The next patient is Felicia, an 18 y/o G2 P1 AB0 who is in the late second trimester of her second pregnancy. Felicia tells you that she has been having severe headaches, and that her feet and ankles are much more swollen than they were in her first pregnancy. Her BP is 160/98, which you know is much higher than normal. You collect a urine specimen from Felicia, and the UA shows protein in her urine. What is the possible diagnosis for Felicia's condition?

_____

4. Another patient, Veronica, brings her baby into the clinic for a four-month checkup. The baby has been closely monitored by the neonatologist because he spent the first month of his life in the neonatal intensive care unit after aspirating early feces before delivery. Which term describes this condition?

_____

Copyright Goodheart-Willcox Co., Inc.
May not be reproduced or posted to a publicly accessible website.

Name _____

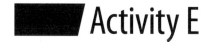 **Activity E   Analyzing Diagnostic-
and Treatment-Related Terms**

Instructions: *Read each of the following scenarios and answer the accompanying questions.*

1. Mary is a 34 y/o G0 P0 who has been unable to get pregnant for more than three years. The physician assistant orders a radiograph imaging procedure to determine whether there is any blockage of Mary's fallopian tubes. What is the name of this procedure?

   _____

2. The PA starts Mary on a medication that stimulates ovulation. What is the classification of this drug?

   _____

3. Six months after this test was performed, Mary makes an appointment to see the PA with c/o amenorrhea for two months. The PA performs a blood test that determines the presence of HCG. Mary's HCG test comes back positive. What is the name of this test, and what does a positive result mean?

   _____

   _____

4. Because Mary is almost 35 y/o, and she has a sister who had a baby with Down syndrome, the PA recommends that Mary have a test in which part of the placenta will be removed and evaluated for chromosomal defects. This test will be performed when Mary is 10–12 weeks pregnant. What is the name of this test?

   _____

5. This test comes back negative. However, because of the risk of genetic conditions in children of older women, the PA recommends another test that will examine the amniotic fluid surrounding the baby. This test will be performed between 15 and 18 weeks gestation. What is the name of this test?

   _____

6. As Mary gets closer to her due date, the baby is turned so that the buttocks are closest to the birth canal. The PA instructs Mary about possibly delivering the baby by an incision through the abdominal wall and uterus. What is the name of this procedure?

   _____

7. One week before Mary's due date, the baby turns in the uterus so that the head is down and ready to go through the birth canal. When Mary is four days past her due date, the PA decides to schedule her and her husband to come into the labor and delivery ward of the hospital. At this time, the PA starts Mary on a medication that will stimulate labor and start her contractions. What is the name of this medication?

   _____

8. During this stage of labor, Mary is fitted with an electronic device that records the baby's heart rate and rhythm. What is the name of this procedure?

   _____

9. Mary's labor starts and her cervix is 100% effaced and dilated. As the baby begins to crown, the obstetrician in the L&D makes an incision into the perineum to prevent tearing. What is the name of this procedure?

   _____

Copyright Goodheart-Willcox Co., Inc.
May not be reproduced or posted to a publicly accessible website.

10. Mary's PA visits her in the postpartum care area of the birthing unit at the hospital. Mary is bonding well with the baby, her colostrum has come in, and the baby is nursing well. Mary and her husband do not want another baby, so they all discuss birth control measures. The PA offers to give Mary a prescription for a medication that will prevent ovulation. What is the classification of this medication?

_____

11. Frances is a 45 y/o G3 P2 AB1 who comes to the gynecologist's office for a follow-up appointment. The nurse practitioner interviews Frances about her health issues. Frances tell her that she is recently divorced and has become sexually active with several partners in the past nine months. The NP asks Frances if she examines her breasts at least once a month to check for any changes. What is this examination called?

_____

12. The NP recommends that Frances have a radiographic examination of her breasts to check for any cancer or other changes. What is the name of this test?

_____

13. Next, the NP prepares Frances for a manual and visual examination of the external and internal female organs. What is the name of this test?

_____

14. Frances tells the NP that she has been having pelvic pain in the area of her right ovary. The NP palpates this area and is concerned about an abnormality. The NP orders a test that uses ultrasonic sound waves to produce an image of a structure in the pelvic cavity. What is the name of this test?

_____

15. Two weeks after these tests, Frances returns to the clinic for a follow-up. The test of her cervical cells came back positive for cervical dysplasia. The NP recommends that Frances tell her sexual partners about this diagnosis. Why is it important for her to notify them of her condition?

_____

_____

_____

16. The NP performs a visual examination of the vagina and cervix with a scope and takes more samples of the tissue of the cervix. What is the name of this procedure?

_____

17. This test comes back positive for cervical cancer. The NP refers Frances to a gynecological oncologist for further evaluation and treatment. The GYN specialist examines Frances' cervix and determines that she needs several procedures. There is one area of diseased tissue on the cervix that she determines can be removed by excising a cone-shaped section. What is the name of this procedure?

_____

18. The GYN specialist decides to remove a small portion of another area on the cervix so that it can be examined under a microscope for further evaluation. What is the name of this procedure?

_____

19. The results of the ultrasound test used to evaluate the right ovary also showed a questionable area on the uterus. The GYN specialist determines that a sample of the endometrial tissue of Frances' uterus needs to be excised so it can be tested for uterine cancer. What is the name of this procedure?

_____

20. These tests come back positive for cervical and uterine cancer. The GYN specialist informs Frances that she will need to have a surgical procedure in which the cervix, uterus, both ovaries, and both fallopian tubes are removed through an incision in the abdomen. What is the name of this procedure?

_____

Copyright Goodheart-Willcox Co., Inc.
May not be reproduced or posted to a publicly accessible website.

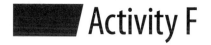 **Activity F   Preparing for Your Future in Healthcare**

Definitions

Instructions: *Using the word parts on pages 438–439, define the following medical terms.*

1. prenatal: _____

2. postnatal:_____

3. antepartum: _____

4. neonatal: _____

5. neonatologist: _____

6. nulligravida: _____

7. primigravida:_____

8. multigravida:_____

9. nullipara:_____

10. primipara: _____

11. multipara: _____

Healthcare Professional Tasks

Instructions: *Use the information on page 466 of your textbook to pair the appropriate healthcare professional with each of the following descriptions or tasks. The healthcare professionals are as follows: obstetrician/ gynecologist, doula, certified nurse midwife (CNM), ultrasound technician. You will use each profession more than once.*

1. takes care of pregnant women from prenatal to postnatal periods: _____

2. can perform surgery:_____

3. graduated from nursing school: _____

4. graduated from medical school: _____

5. generally has routine (or set) hours for his or her job: _____

6. generally does not have routine (or set) hours for his or her job:_____

7. may be involved in at-home births: _____

8. performs diagnostic tests that are ordered by other healthcare professionals: _____

9. generally requires more schooling than the other listed professionals: _____

Copyright Goodheart-Willcox Co., Inc.
May not be reproduced or posted to a publicly accessible website.

Chapter 14 Practice Test

Term Identification

Instructions: *Identify the term that corresponds to each of the following descriptions.*

1. the surgical removal of a breast lump: _____

2. the state of a false pregnancy: _____

3. a hernia or swelling of a fallopian tube: _____

4. surgical repair of the vulva: _____

Medical Terms and Definitions

Instructions: *Break down each of the following medical terms into its word parts (prefix, root word, combining vowel, and suffix if used). Then define each term.*

1. mastoptosis

   Breakdown: _____

   Define: _____

2. mastopexy

   Breakdown: _____

   Define: _____

3. perimetritis

   Breakdown: _____

   Define: _____

4. dysmenorrhea

   Breakdown: _____

   Define: _____

5. endocervicitis

   Breakdown: _____

   Define: _____

6. colpoperineorrhaphy

   Breakdown: _____

   Define: _____

Copyright Goodheart-Willcox Co., Inc.
May not be reproduced or posted to a publicly accessible website.

Name _____

Review

Instructions: *Answer the following questions.*

1. Which organ of the female reproductive system is also considered part of the endocrine system?

   _____

2. What is the singular form of the term *ova*?

   _____

3. In which structure does conception generally take place?

   _____

4. In most women, which way does the uterus lean?

   _____

5. What is the anatomical term for the birth canal?

   _____

6. What part of the uterus is shed during the monthly menstrual cycle?

   _____

7. Where is the hymen located?

   _____

8. Which term describes the innermost "lips" of the vagina?

   _____

9. What is another term for the vaginal opening?

   _____

10. What type of tissue surrounds the mammary glands?

    _____

11. Which term describes a zygote at three days after conception?

    _____

12. Which term describes a birth that occurs before 37 weeks of gestation?

    _____

13. Which term describes the fluid that surrounds the fetus?

    _____

14. What helps move the baby out of the uterus and into the birth canal?

    _____

15. What is the difference between *effacement* and *dilation*?

    _____

16. Why do identical twins share DNA?

    _____

Copyright Goodheart-Willcox Co., Inc.
May not be reproduced or posted to a publicly accessible website.

Matching

Instructions: *Match each of the following diseases or conditions with the correct meaning.*

1. _____ a toxic condition of pregnancy characterized by HTN, albuminuria, and edema

2. _____ hernia of the bladder that protrudes through the vaginal wall

3. _____ erythroblastosis fetalis

4. _____ complication of pregnancy in which the zygote implants outside of the uterus

5. _____ pain in the breast that may signal a noncancerous breast condition

6. _____ condition in which the placenta implants at the lower end of the uterus

7. _____ excessively heavy menstrual flow

8. _____ herniation of the rectum through the posterior vaginal wall

9. _____ loss of a fetus before it is viable

10. _____ life-threatening complication of pregnancy characterized by HTN and seizures

A. miscarriage
B. rectocele
C. placenta previa
D. eclampsia
E. cystocele
F. hemolytic disease of the newborn
G. ectopic pregnancy
H. menorrhagia
I. preeclampsia
J. mastalgia

Copyright Goodheart-Willcox Co., Inc.
May not be reproduced or posted to a publicly accessible website.